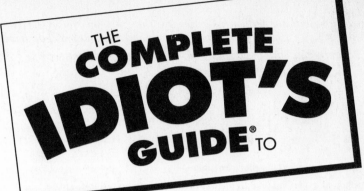

THE COMPLETE IDIOT'S GUIDE® TO

Type 2 Diabetes

by Mayer B. Davidson, M.D., and Debra L. Gordon

ALPHA

A member of Penguin Group (USA) Inc.

Dr. Davidson dedicates this book to the millions of patients with type 2 diabetes in the fervent hope that the information contained herein will help them avoid the terrible complications that diabetes can cause.

Debra Gordon dedicates this book to her husband, Keith, without whom nothing is possible.

ALPHA BOOKS

Published by the Penguin Group

Penguin Group (USA) Inc., 375 Hudson Street, New York, New York 10014, U.S.A.

Penguin Group (Canada), 10 Alcorn Avenue, Toronto, Ontario, Canada M4V 3B2 (a division of Pearson Penguin Canada Inc.)

Penguin Books Ltd, 80 Strand, London WC2R 0RL, England

Penguin Ireland, 25 St Stephen's Green, Dublin 2, Ireland (a division of Penguin Books Ltd)

Penguin Group (Australia), 250 Camberwell Road, Camberwell, Victoria 3124, Australia (a division of Pearson Australia Group Pty Ltd)

Penguin Books India Pvt Ltd, 11 Community Centre, Panchsheel Park, New Delhi - 110 017, India

Penguin Group (NZ), Cnr Airborne and Rosedale Roads, Albany, Auckland, New Zealand (a division of Pearson New Zealand Ltd)

Penguin Books (South Africa) (Pty) Ltd, 24 Sturdee Avenue, Rosebank, Johannesburg 2196, South Africa

Penguin Books Ltd, Registered Offices: 80 Strand, London WC2R 0RL, England

International Standard Book Number: 1-59257-409-2
Library of Congress Catalog Card Number: 2005929444

07 06 05   8 7 6 5 4 3 2 1

Interpretation of the printing code: The rightmost number of the first series of numbers is the year of the book's printing; the rightmost number of the second series of numbers is the number of the book's printing. For example, a printing code of 05-1 shows that the first printing occurred in 2005.

Printed in the United States of America

Note: This publication contains the opinions and ideas of its authors. It is intended to provide helpful and informative material on the subject matter covered. It is sold with the understanding that the authors and publisher are not engaged in rendering professional services in the book. If the reader requires personal assistance or advice, a competent professional should be consulted.

The authors and publisher specifically disclaim any responsibility for any liability, loss, or risk, personal or otherwise, which is incurred as a consequence, directly or indirectly, of the use and application of any of the contents of this book.

Most Alpha books are available at special quantity discounts for bulk purchases for sales promotions, premiums, fundraising, or educational use. Special books, or book excerpts, can also be created to fit specific needs.

For details, write: Special Markets, Alpha Books, 375 Hudson Street, New York, NY 10014.

Publisher: *Marie Butler-Knight*
Product Manager: *Phil Kitchel*
Senior Managing Editor: *Jennifer Bowles*
Senior Acquisitions Editor: *Mike Sanders*
Development Editor: *Ginny Bess Munroe*
Production Editor: *Megan Douglass*

Copy Editor: *Jan Zoya*
Cartoonist: *Richard King*
Cover/Book Designer: *Trina Wurst*
Indexer: *Angie Bess*
Proofreading: *Mary Hunt*
Layout: *Angela Calvert Johnson*

Contents at a Glance

Contents

Foreword

It is not happenstance that accounts for the enormous amount of press that has been given to diabetes in the past few years. It is clear from a compelling body of evidence that the decade of the '90s witnessed an explosion of diabetes, elevating this disease to true epidemic status. It is the epidemic of our time, and its excess morbidity, healthcare costs, and mortality are well-documented. It is fair to say, however, that physicians and scientists have not been idle in the face of this growing problem. On the contrary, there have been extraordinary advances made in our understanding of virtually every aspect of this disease. We understand a great deal about the underlying causes for all the major types of diabetes, including type 1, type 2, and gestational diabetes. We have gained important insights on the complex genetics of this disease, and on the metabolic defects that occur in liver, muscle, and fat which drive the hyperglycemia and abnormal lipids of diabetes. Insulin resistance is now understood to be a systemic condition accompanied by changes that make an affected person more prone to high blood pressure, blood clot formation, inflammation, and higher levels of blood sugar and blood fats. It is this collection of risk factors in the setting of insulin resistance that result in the higher rates of cardiovascular disease like heart attacks and strokes in diabetes. In many ways, this is good news that we understand so much of the cellular, genetic, and molecular events that lead to many of the outcomes we experience in diabetes. It is even better news for the over 18 million persons with diabetes that we can design treatment strategies that will actually prevent the onset or delay the progression of many of these serious complications. We can say with certainty what the goals are for blood sugar, blood pressure, and blood fats, both cholesterol and triglycerides, in order to prevent these outcomes. The lessons we have learned about lifestyle changes, the powerful new medications, the new delivery systems and convenient monitoring devices can be used to good advantage in people with diabetes. Thus, it is nothing short of disappointing that so few people are achieving the required treatment goals and preventing the outcomes in diabetes. Why have we accomplished such poor translation of this abundant fundamental knowledge about diabetes into clinical results in our patients?

While there is no simple answer to this question, it is clear that diabetes must be managed primarily by patients themselves, who must be capable of making the daily choices regarding nutrition, physical activity, medication adjustment, and stress management that affect the status of their diabetes. They must be prepared to regularly interact with the other members of the diabetes team, including the diabetes educator, the physician, the nutritionist, the pharmacist, among others. They must have a strong foundation of basic understanding about the many aspects of this disease, including the physiology, the signs and symptoms, the meaning of high and low levels of glucose, the meaning of glycated hemoglobin, or A1C, the significance of trace amounts of protein in the urine, the difference between the calories per gram of carbohydrate versus fat. These same persons must understand how metformin is different from a sulfonylurea, what an insulin sensitizer is, and what the various types of insulin do to blood sugar levels over short and over long periods of time. Since there is virtually no aspect of a person's physical or psychological being unaffected by diabetes, there is a great deal to understand. As challenging as it seems, it is unavoidable that the patient must become an expert in the management of her disease. This requires not just a familiarity, but some mastery of the basics of diabetes and the most effective strategies of self-care. It does not stop there. A person needs to understand the policies, practices and procedures of insurance companies who cover the costs of goods and services used by people with diabetes. People with diabetes must understand the implications of major health legislation like the Medicare Modernization Act and how it will affect their individual access to various types of coverage and care or those of loved ones.

It is a real challenge to assemble and express this vast and complex mix of issues in a way that takes the mystery and confusion out of the various discussions about diabetes. This book takes on precisely this challenge and scores a major achievement. The authors combine their different experience and perspectives on this disease to produce information that the average person can relate to and understand. They have reduced complicated scientific and biologic concepts to a practical conversation that can occur with relative ease between patients and any members of the diabetes healthcare team. What is more, the book is organized in ways that allow a person to go directly to the sections that are most applicable and pressing for their individual circumstance. With comprehensive, cutting-edge discussions of all of the major clinically-relevant areas of diabetes, whether cause or consequence, this is truly a complete guide. It is an excellent general reference source about the broad range of topics encountered in diabetes care, including a much-needed segment on what clinical trials are and how they have contributed to improvements in patient care. The authors have included intermittent short segments called "Bet You Didn't Know" to introduce special items of interest to all persons with diabetes. Just reading these alone makes this book a valuable guide. This is a book that will stimulate conversations about diabetes between friends and family, and between the patient and healthcare providers. While it does an admirable job of answering a lot of questions, my expectation is that it will prompt the asking of a great deal more. That is a good thing, actually. Otherwise, I do not know how the "idiot" for whom this book is intended will ever rise to the level of an informed, empowered, and activated patient advocate so essential in stemming the tide of this epidemic among us. This is a must read for all persons ready to assume greater control and assure better outcomes in diabetes. Surely any idiot would want that.

James R. Gavin III, M.D., Ph.D.
Chair, National Diabetes Education Program
Past President, American Diabetes Association
Professor of Medicine
Emory University School of Medicine
Atlanta, Georgia

Introduction

Our country, indeed, the entire developed world, is facing a health epidemic of frightening proportions. It's not caused by a virus, a bacteria, or anything you can catch. Instead, this burgeoning epidemic is the result of our modern lifestyles, lives in which high-fat, sugar-filled food is everywhere we turn, in which we can go days without doing anything more strenuous than turning the key in a car or flipping channels with a remote.

We're talking, of course, about type 2 diabetes, which affects more than 16 million Americans. How serious is the epidemic? Just consider that one in three Americans born in 2000 will develop diabetes during their lifetime. Left unchecked, this will lead to a crisis in our healthcare system and the health of our population that has never before been seen.

For diabetes is not simply a disease of high blood sugar, but a leading cause of blindness, limb amputations, nerve system disorders, and heart disease in the country.

Despite the huge numbers of people who already have diabetes, however, much of the available information about living with type 2 diabetes is contradictory and confusing. That's why we've written *The Complete Idiot's Guide to Type 2 Diabetes.* We wanted to provide a clear, easy-to-understand guide to type 2 diabetes and its complications so you can learn to control your disease—instead of allowing *it* to control *you.*

In this book, you'll learn how to put together a healthcare team, how to handle your diabetes in the workplace, how to prevent and, if necessary, manage complications. We'll help you work through some very personal issues with your diabetes, like its effect on your sex life, as well as some very public issues—like how and when to tell the people in your life about your disease.

Most important, we'll give you the information and the tools you need to stay motivated to lose weight, eat right, exercise, and control your blood glucose, blood pressure, and cholesterol levels. For in the end, you are ultimately the one in charge of your disease—not your doctor.

By taking a proactive approach to your diabetes, you can turn what could be a devastating killer into a manageable, chronic disease that, while it will require certain changes in your life, won't interfere with your life itself.

How to Use This Book

There's a lot to cover with a condition as all encompassing as diabetes. We've tried to break it down into manageable chunks for you:

In **Part 1, "Diabetes Uncovered,"** we briefly discuss emerging diabetes epidemic and how to cope with your diagnosis. Then we give you an overview of what's happening in your body when you have diabetes, explaining the importance of balance in a healthy body.

In **Part 2, "Traveling the Treatment Trail,"** we focus on how you need to treat your diabetes. For instance, we show you how to put together a treatment team in Chapter 4, and the kind of lifestyle changes you need to make in terms of exercise and diet. But we do more than just *tell* you you should do; we also give you helpful hints for everything from easy ways to get 30 minutes a day of physical activity to how to eat out in Chinese restaurants and not send your blood sugar levels skyrocketing. We also help you understand how the medications your doctor has prescribed work in your body, the best ways to take them, and which might be better for you.

Once you understand how to treat your diabetes, it's time to talk about managing your diabetes while integrating it into your life in **Part 3, "Daily Living with Diabetes."** That's why we have chapters on blood glucose meters (including one you wear as a watch), the affect of stress, sleep and sickness on your diabetes (bet you didn't know a good night's sleep can do wonders for your blood sugar), and we even tackle a topic most people shy away from—sex. Finally, for the younger women out there, we tell you what you need to know to get pregnant and have a healthy pregnancy and baby—despite your diabetes.

In **Part 4, "Avoiding Complications,"** things get serious. That's where we show you what could happen to you if you don't manage your blood sugar levels, and why the diabetes itself might be the least of your problems. But, rather than dwell on the gloom and doom, we also provide a lot of helpful advice for avoiding these worst-case scenarios, whether its kidney disease, blindness, diabetic neuropathy, or limb amputation.

And in **Part 5, "A Glimpse into the Future,"** we let you know what's coming. From new drugs to stem cell transplants that might actually cure diabetes, we cover it all.

Extra Help

As you read you'll find boxes scattered throughout the chapters. Each type of box contains different information that you'll find interesting and useful in different situations.

Bet You Didn't Know

These boxes contain stuff we thought was interesting that we "bet you didn't know." Though this information probably won't help you manage your diabetes, it might help you better understand your disease and its treatments.

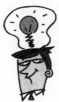

Sugar Sense

If there's a better way to take a drug, a certain type of mineral that's better than another, or a unique way we've found to manage your disease, you'll find it in these boxes.

MedLingo

Medicalese can be hard to understand. So we've provided you with at-a-glance definitions for many of the more complicated terms we use throughout the book.

Warning

As the name implies, these boxes point out things you need to know to manage your diabetes and you're your medications safely and effectively.

Acknowledgments

This book was most definitely a team effort, and we want to thank the people at Alpha books for their patience and guidance throughout the process, particularly acquisitions editor Mike Sanders and developmental editor Ginny Bess.

Debra wants to give particular thanks to Mayer B. Davidson, M.D. He carved out huge chunks of time from his busy schedule to work on this book, patiently explaining nuances of physiology and diabetes to Debra without any criticism. She would also like to thank her agent, Marilyn Allen, for bringing this project to her attention, and Kathleen Weaver, who has type 2 diabetes and who was very generous in sharing her own experiences with the disease. And, of course, her ever-patient, ever-loving husband, Keith, and her sons, Callum, Iain, and Jonathan, for understanding why Mom is always, yes, always, in front of her computer.

For his part, Mayer was very impressed with Debra's ability to capture and describe so much information so quickly, and, for the most part, so accurately. We also gratefully acknowledge the expert contributions to Chapter 15 on workplace discrimination from Michael A. Greene, an attorney who specializes in employment discrimination. He is a past Chairman of the Board of Directors of the American Diabetes

Association (1993-1994) and has led the efforts to counter employment discrimination for people with diabetes. He has been the lead volunteer attorney for the American Diabetes Association in many of their groundbreaking cases. Mr. Greene is a partner in the law firm of Rosenthal & Greene, 1001 Southwest Fifth Avenue, Suite 1907, Portland, OR, 97204, (503) 228-3015.

Trademarks

All terms mentioned in this book that are known to be or are suspected of being trademarks or service marks have been appropriately capitalized. Alpha Books and Penguin Group (USA) Inc. cannot attest to the accuracy of this information. Use of a term in this book should not be regarded as affecting the validity of any trademark or service mark.

Part 1

Type 2 Diabetes Uncovered

In this part of the book, you'll learn why so many people are getting type 2 diabetes and how it differs from other types of diabetes. You'll get a good understanding of how to cope with your diagnosis and share your news with your family and friends. In Chapter 3, you'll learn about the physical aspects of diabetes—how it occurs, the parts of your body involved, and why it happens.

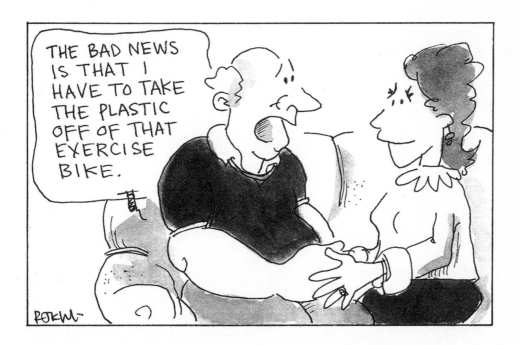

An Emerging Epidemic

In This Chapter

- ◆ Diabetes by the numbers
- ◆ Why more people have diabetes
- ◆ Type 2 diabetes
- ◆ Type 1 diabetes
- ◆ Gestational diabetes
- ◆ Diabetes in women

Maybe you've just been told that you have diabetes or are at risk of developing diabetes. Maybe a close friend or family member has just been diagnosed with the disease.

And so you have questions. Lots of questions. Relax. We answer them all right here. First, though, we need to talk about the growing numbers of people with diabetes, and why their numbers keep rising. We need to understand why public health officials call diabetes an *epidemic*—a word they don't use lightly. This is what we discuss in this chapter.

Who Has It?

It is estimated that one in three Americans born in 2000 will develop diabetes during his or her lifetime. But that figure is just the tip of the iceberg. Overall, the numbers that describe today's diabetes *epidemic* are staggering:

MedLingo

An **epidemic** is a widespread outbreak of a disease that affects many people at one time. It can also describe a disease, not by the number of people who have it, but by how fast it is growing. Diabetes fulfills both of these criteria.

- More than 18 million Americans have diabetes.

- One in five people (20 percent) over the age of 65 has diabetes.

- The number of American adults with diagnosed diabetes has increased 61 percent since 1991, and will more than double by 2050.

- 5.2 million Americans who have diabetes don't even know they have it.

- Type 2 diabetes, which is linked to obesity and physical inactivity, accounts for 90 to 95 percent of all cases of diabetes.

Bet You Didn't Know

Diabetes takes a tremendous cost not only in terms of human lives, but also in terms of our pocketbooks. Diabetes costs the nation nearly $132 billion a year, making it one of the most expensive diseases in our healthcare system. The average health costs for a person with diabetes is more than $13,000 a year, compared to about $2,500 for someone without the disease.

Just What *Is* Diabetes Anyway?

Diabetes is much more complex than simply a disease in which your blood sugar gets too high. Basically, people with diabetes don't make enough *insulin*, a *hormone* that helps your cells take up sugar for energy, and/or they have problems responding to the insulin their body does make.

Insulin enables glucose to enter muscle and fat cells, where it can be used as energy and stored for future use in a form called glycogen. Between meals and overnight, the liver produces glucose. Insulin plays a role there by ensuring that the liver produces just the right amount of glucose to maintain normal blood sugar levels.

In type 1 diabetes, the body makes no insulin; in type 2 diabetes, the situation is more complicated. Some people with the disease have a hard time using the insulin they make, so they wind up making extra insulin. Others with the disease don't make enough insulin to maintain normal blood sugar levels.

When diabetes isn't controlled, fats and sugar from the food you eat build up in your blood and, over time, can significantly damage blood vessels and other organs. This damage, in turn, can lead to many other conditions and complications, including blindness, heart disease, nerve damage, and kidney failure. It can even make you more likely to die from something as common as the flu. We talk more about these complications later.

MedLingo

Hormones are chemical messengers that provide instructions to your cells. **Insulin** is a hormone secreted by specialized cells in the pancreas. Its role is to maintain normal blood sugar levels, to keep fat stored in fat cells, and to make sure that protein is used to build muscles.

Why Do So Many People Have Diabetes?

Between 1980 and 2002, the number of Americans with diabetes more than doubled—from 5.8 million to 13.3 million. Much of that increase has come in just the past decade or so, with the number of American adults with diagnosed diabetes, including women with *gestational diabetes*, increasing 61 percent since 1991.

Why the jump? Well, one of the best ways to explain it is with the story of the Pima Indians.

MedLingo

Gestational diabetes is actually glucose intolerance that occurs during pregnancy. Glucose intolerance is defined as glucose levels during an oral glucose tolerance test that falls between normal and diabetes. However, since the fetus of pregnant women with glucose intolerance can have so many problems, this condition is called "gestational diabetes." The glucose intolerance often goes away once the baby is born but women who have had gestational diabetes are much more likely to get type 2 diabetes later on in life.

Pima Indians: The Canary in the Mine

You probably never heard of the Pima Indians, but they're famous among diabetes researchers. They're also a perfect example of how the way we live affects our likelihood of getting diabetes.

The National Institute for Diabetes, Digestive, and Kidney Diseases (NIDDK) has been studying the Pima Indians in Arizona and Mexico for more than 30 years. It is through these studies that we now know that obesity is a major risk factor in the development of diabetes. Why? Because half of all adult Pima Indians have diabetes, and 95 percent of those with diabetes are overweight. This finding, in turn, has led to the "thrifty gene" theory to explain the prevalence of diabetes in the Western world today.

From Thrifty Gene to Obesity

The thrifty gene theory works like this: The Pima Indians, like most humans, have traditionally been a people who relied on farming, hunting, and fishing for sustenance for thousands of years. Sometimes there was plenty of food, sometimes not so much. Over time, their genetic makeup changed so that their bodies learned to hang on to every calorie (in the form of stored fat) that came its way because they never knew when another famine would strike.

Fast forward to the present. With food everywhere in our world today (at least in industrialized countries), and physical activity a minor part of our lives, starvation is hardly a problem. But our bodies are still in the feast-or-famine mode, still trained to hang onto every calorie for dear life. Therefore, we get fat.

Scientists can see this most clearly with the Pimas of Arizona because until World War II, they continued to live in their old ways. After the war, their traditional way of life was disrupted when they began living on a reservation.

That's when their diet changed to one containing high-fat and high-sugar foods. At the same time, their physical activity levels significantly decreased. For instance, with running water available, they didn't have to haul water from wells, and with cars and pickup trucks, they didn't have to walk much anymore. Their weight—and the number of Pimas with diabetes—ballooned.

How do we know to blame what they ate and their lack of activity? Well, compare the Arizonan Pimas to their Mexican cousins. In the mountains of Mexico, where the Pimas are genetically similar to their Arizona relatives, the traditional life still holds sway. Even though the Mexican Pimas take in more calories than the Arizonans, diabetes is rare, and being overweight is even more unusual. That's likely because they get significantly more physical activity and eat diets higher in fiber and lower in sugar or fat than their American cousins.

The moral of the Pima Indian story? Even though you may be genetically programmed to get diabetes, your environment, or how you live, makes a big difference and can modify your genetic risk.

But I'm Not a Pima Indian; Why Do I Have Diabetes?

The Pimas are just an extreme example of what's happening to all of us today. Scientists think that most people, to one extent or another, have some version of this "thrifty gene." Just consider that today, about 64 percent of Americans are overweight, and 30 percent are *very* overweight, or obese. In fact, the World Health Organization has declared being overweight one of the top 10 health risks in the world, and one of the top 5 in developed nations (like ours).

You're considered overweight if you have a *body mass index*, or BMI, between 25 and 30, and you're considered obese if you have a BMI of 30 or more.

Being overweight is huge risk factor for type 2 diabetes, the most common form of diabetes and the type we're focusing on in this book.

These days, knowing your weight isn't enough. You also need to know what your BMI, or body mass index, is. It's easy enough to figure out. Start with your weight in pounds divided by your height in inches squared (in other words, multiply your height by itself). Now multiply that whole result by 703. *Voilà!* Your BMI. The following table shows what it means:

MedLingo

The **body mass index (BMI)** is a measurement used to classify people according to their weight (underweight, normal, overweight, obese), taking height into account.

Relationship Between BMI and Weight Status

BMI	Weight Status
Below 18.5	Underweight
18.5 – 24.9	Normal
25.0 – 29.9	Overweight
30.0 and above	Obese

Source: Centers for Disease Control

MedLingo

The **pancreas** is an organ whose main function is to secrete enzymes into the small intestine to help digest food. About 1 percent of the pancreas also secretes hormones into the bloodstream. Insulin is the most important hormone secreted.

It seems that in people who are overweight (and more than 80 percent of people with type 2 diabetes *are*), their muscle cells, where glucose (or sugar) enters and is broken down, simply don't respond as well to insulin. So sugar builds up in their blood. High levels of blood sugar send signals to your *pancreas* to make more and more insulin. Eventually, however, the pancreas gives up, and cuts back on the amount of insulin it's making. Boom! Diabetes.

Why Are Americans So Fat?

Lots of reasons. Let's start with the availability of food. There's food in department stores, food in gas stations, food at nearly every social gathering we attend. But it's not just the food itself that's the problem; it's the *kind* of food we eat today.

Much of what we purchase and consume is processed food, filled with fat, sugar, and salt. Instead of water, we drink high calorie sodas and fruit drinks. Instead of a piece of fruit, we munch on potato chips for a snack. Instead of a high-fiber, low-calorie salad, we hit the drive-thru for a burger and fries. Which brings us to the next reason we're so fat: the supersizing of America.

Just consider that 20 years ago, the hamburger and french fries now sold as the children's meal at McDonalds was actually the normal-size meal that most customers ordered. Then restaurateurs figured out that Americans were more interested in quantity and value than anything else, and began supersizing everything. Today, the 7-Eleven Double Gulp, a 64-oz. soda, contains nearly 800 calories, 10 times the size of a Coke when it was introduced. This provides more than one third of the daily calories most people require! (And it explains why car manufacturers have increased the size of cup holders in American cars.)

Bet You Didn't Know

Between 1977 and 1995, Americans increased the amount of calories they ate and drank on a daily basis by nearly 200 calories per day. We went from 1,876 calories to 2,043 calories. Since it takes about 3,600 calories to equal one pound, that's an extra 16.9 pounds a year you're packing on if you haven't upped your physical activity enough to burn those extra 200 calories.

All this food wouldn't be so terrible, however, if we were expending the energy to use up those thousands of calories we're taking in these days, say, by chopping down trees, plowing a field, or hauling fishing nets.

Instead, we're sitting behind computers, e-mailing the person in the next cubicle instead of getting up to talk, clicking the remote at the TV so that we don't have to get up and change channels, and hitting drive-thrus for everything from food to money to dry cleaning. Today, less than half of Americans get the recommended 30 minutes a day or more of physical activity. Most jobs are sedentary, and manufacturers continue to come up with one labor-saving device after another (consider the dishwasher, riding lawn mower and leaf blower, for example).

Plus, tasks that used to help us burn calories—yard work, housekeeping, painting the shutters—are now more likely to be hired out. You can even hire someone to walk your dog!

We cover more about the impact of exercise on diabetes later—in terms of both preventing and treating it. But for now, just know that that sitting on your duff all day can do as much to increase your risk of diabetes, and make any existing case of diabetes worse, as eating a box of donuts.

Deconstructing Type 2 Diabetes

Never heard of type 2 diabetes? Don't worry. For years, it was called "adult onset" diabetes or noninsulin dependent diabetes. Neither of those monikers is accurate, however, for a variety of reasons. For one, children are increasingly developing type 2 diabetes. For another, about 40 percent of people with this form of diabetes eventually require daily injections of insulin to treat their disease; hardly a "noninsulin dependent" form of diabetes!

Generally, in type 2 diabetes, your body still makes some insulin. It just can't respond to the insulin very effectively. It's kind of like filling up your car with a full tank of gas, but because the gas line is kinked, your car's engine doesn't get the fuel that it needs to run. Before a person gets type 2 diabetes, the pancreas has to produce extra insulin to get around that kink in the gas line. Eventually, however, your body gets tired of producing the extra insulin and begins shutting down production.

Who Gets It?

Overall, between 90 and 95 percent of all people with diabetes have type 2 diabetes; and the growing epidemic of diabetes in this country is related to the growing number of people with type 2 diabetes.

You're more likely to develop type 2 diabetes if you're overweight, 45 or older, exercise less than three times a week, have a family history of diabetes, have high blood pressure, have high levels of *triglycerides*, or had diabetes while you were pregnant (gestational diabetes).

MedLingo

Triglycerides are a form of fat carried in the bloodstream and stored in fat tissue.

You're also more likely to get type 2 diabetes if you're African American, Hispanic, Asian, Native American, or hail from a Pacific Island like Guam or Hawaii.

Slowly Developing Symptoms

As we noted earlier, about five million people have type 2 diabetes and don't even know they have it. How can this be? Well, the symptoms of very high blood sugars occur in only a minority of patients with type 2 diabetes who have very high blood glucose levels. These symptoms include the following:

- ◆ Unusual thirst (which leads to the next symptom)
- ◆ Frequent urination
- ◆ Unintended weight loss
- ◆ Blurred vision

- ◆ Frequent infections
- ◆ Slow healing of wounds or sores

Sugar Sense

If you're 45 or older, or are younger than 45 but are overweight and have one or more of the risk factors for diabetes, you should have your blood sugar levels tested.

But most people don't develop *any* symptoms early on. That's why 75 percent of all cases of type 2 diabetes are discovered during routine testing. However, if blood glucose levels remain high over years, they eventually cause the eye, kidney and nerve complications of diabetes described later in the book.

Don't Forget These Other Types

Although we're focusing on type 2 diabetes in this book (and, after this chapter, any reference to "diabetes" will be a reference to type 2 diabetes), it is helpful to understand the two other main types of diabetes: type 1 and gestational diabetes, and how they differ from the type of diabetes you have.

Type 1 Diabetes: Sudden and Dramatic

Type 1 diabetes, which used to be called "juvenile" diabetes, represents the minority of diabetes cases, but it is often the most difficult to treat and the one most likely to cause complications, primarily because people with the disease develop it so early in their lives.

Type 1 diabetes is actually an *autoimmune disease*, which means that the immune system, the part of body that normally protects us from disease by attacking germs like viruses and bacteria, goes haywire and begins attacking normal cells that belong to us. With type 1 diabetes, the immune system attacks and destroys special cells in the pancreas called *beta cells* that make insulin. Thus, the pancreas is unable to produce much, if any, insulin. Someone with type 1 diabetes has to take insulin several times every day.

MedLingo

An **autoimmune disease** occurs when the immune system begins destroying normal, healthy cells. Autoimmune diseases include lupus, multiple sclerosis, and rheumatoid arthritis.

Beta cells are specialized cells within the pancreas that make insulin. They are located in structures distributed throughout the pancreas called the islets of Langerhans (they looked like islands to the German physician who first described them in the nineteenth century) and make up only 1 percent of the pancreas.

No one really knows why the immune system suddenly turns on the pancreatic beta cells. Although only people with a certain genetic background get type 1 diabetes, this genetic background is present in almost half of the population. Why only a few individuals within this genetic background get type 1 diabetes is unclear. The reason might be related to a virus or other environmental factors such as toxins. No one really knows. Although type 1 diabetes usually occurs in children and young adults, particularly adolescents, it can occur at any age.

Gestational Diabetes: Only During Pregnancy

About 4 out of every 100 pregnant women who never had diabetes develop a form of the disease called gestational diabetes. Women with this condition have blood sugars between normal and levels high enough to diagnose diabetes in those who are not pregnant. These higher-than-normal blood sugars can cause problems during delivery and during the baby's first few weeks of life.

Gestational diabetes is caused when the pancreas can't keep up with the extra demands placed on it during pregnancy. As the *placenta* (the lining between the developing fetus and the mother's uterus) grows, it produces larger and larger amounts of the hormones that make it difficult for the insulin produced in the mother to work. In most women, the pancreas can keep up with this extra demand, producing enough insulin to keep blood sugars normal. However, in about 4 percent of women, the pancreas can't produce enough extra insulin, resulting in high levels of blood sugar, a condition called *hyperglycemia*.

MedLingo

Hyperglycemia occurs when your blood glucose levels get too high.

Testing for Gestational Diabetes

Today, nearly all obstetricians test for gestational diabetes between the twenty-fourth and twenty-eighth week of pregnancy. The mother-to-be is asked to drink a sugary liquid in the doctor's office. After an hour, her blood is tested to see if her blood sugar levels are too high.

If they are too high, she returns for an oral glucose tolerance test. In this test, she fasts overnight. In the morning, a blood sample is drawn before she drinks an even more sugary liquid than she drank for the first test. Additional blood is drawn each hour for the next three hours and her blood sugar levels are tested.

Treating Gestational Diabetes

In the majority of women, gestational diabetes is treated with diet and exercise. However, in some women, insulin might be required, especially toward the end of pregnancy.

It is important to treat gestational diabetes. That's because the extra glucose in the mother's system crosses the placenta and goes into the baby. This can cause an overly large baby, which can result in a difficult delivery. Babies exposed to too much insulin in utero are also at risk of low blood sugar and other problems after they're born, and have a much higher risk of becoming obese and developing type 2 diabetes themselves later in life.

Although gestational diabetes disappears soon after the baby is born, it is an important indicator of risk for type 2 diabetes later in life. Women who have had gestational diabetes have a 20 to 50 percent chance of developing type 2 diabetes within 5 to 15 years of their pregnancy. If you have had gestational diabetes, the best way to avoid developing type 2 diabetes later is to maintain a healthy weight and to exercise regularly.

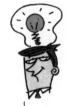

Sugar Sense

You may be able to prevent gestational diabetes during pregnancy by doing the following:

♦ **Eating a healthy diet.** That means a diet high in fruits and vegetables, low in simple carbohydrates like cakes, cookies, and chips, low in saturated fat, and high in healthy protein, like fish, chicken, and soy products.

♦ **Getting regular exercise.** This includes walking, yoga, swimming, or exercise classes designed especially for pregnant women. As always, get your doctor's okay before beginning any exercise program.

♦ **Maintaining a healthy weight throughout your pregnancy.** Women who were of normal weight when they got pregnant should gain 25 to 35 pounds; those who were overweight or obese should gain 15 to 25 pounds.

Other Specific Types of Diabetes

A small percentage of diabetes cases are caused by a variety of other causes, including the following:

♦ Genetic defects in the cells responsible for the production of or response to insulin

♦ Diseases that affect the pancreas, such as cystic fibrosis, hemochromatosis (a condition in which too much iron builds up in the tissues), pancreatitis (an inflammation of the pancreas, usually brought on by gall stones or too much alcohol), or pancreatic cancer

♦ Hormonal diseases, including Cushing's syndrome (when the body produces too much of a certain kind of steroid called glucocorticoids), acromegaly (when the body produces too much growth hormone), and pheochromocytoma (when the body produces too much adrenaline)

♦ Certain drugs or chemicals, such as glucocorticoids.

> **CAUTION**
>
> **Warning** _____
>
> The following drugs can contribute to or result in the development of diabetes. Make sure that all of your doctors know if you're taking one or more of these drugs, and be extra vigilant about recognizing the signs of diabetes.
>
> ◆ **Nicotinic acid,** often used to treat high cholesterol
>
> ◆ **Glucocorticoids,** such as prednisone, dexamethasone, and hydrocortisone, often used to treat asthma and other immune system diseases
>
> ◆ **Dilantin,** often used to prevent seizures

Gender Differences: Diabetes in Women

Diabetes, like most diseases, is most definitely not gender neutral. It can behave differently in women, and even has some higher risks of complications for women than for men.

For instance …

◆ Women without diabetes have fewer heart problems than men. However, if you have diabetes, your risk of heart disease is equal to that of men with diabetes. While a man with diabetes is twice as likely to die of a heart attack as a man without diabetes, a woman with diabetes is four to five times more likely to die of a heart attack than a woman without diabetes.

> **CAUTION**
>
> **Warning** _____
>
> Women with diabetes tend to have more bladder infections and yeast infections than women without the disease. Both infections are a sign that your blood sugar levels may be too high.

◆ Women with diabetes have a shorter life expectancy than women without diabetes.

◆ Women with diabetes are 50 percent more likely to develop *diabetic ketoacidosis*, a diabetic coma resulting from poorly controlled diabetes and high blood glucose levels, than men with the disease.

◆ Women with diabetes are 7.6 times more likely to suffer *peripheral vascular disease (PVD)* than women without diabetes.

Of course, the greatest risk to women with diabetes occurs during pregnancy, when the condition can cause complications to both mother and baby. We tell you more about diabetes during pregnancy in Chapter 14.

MedLingo

Diabetic ketoacidosis (DKA) is an emergency condition in which extremely high blood glucose levels, along with a severe lack of insulin, result in the breakdown of body fat for energy and an accumulation of ketones in the blood and urine. Because ketones are weak acids, the body becomes too acidic. Signs of DKA are nausea and vomiting, stomach pain, fruity breath odor, and rapid breathing, along with the symptoms of very high blood sugars mentioned earlier, such as increased thirst, frequent urination, and blurred vision. Untreated DKA can lead to coma and death.

Peripheral vascular disease is a condition in which the blood vessels in the legs narrow, causing pain. Left untreated, it can lead to amputation. It also increases one's risk for heart disease and stroke.

The Least You Need to Know

◆ Diabetes is a growing epidemic in this country.

◆ The growing numbers of overweight and obese children and adults are directly linked to the growing number of people with diabetes.

◆ There are three primary types of diabetes: type 1, in which the body makes no insulin; type 2, in which the body doesn't respond to the insulin it produces very well, and eventually can't continue producing the extra insulin demanded; and gestational diabetes, which occurs during pregnancy.

◆ Diabetes can also be caused by some medical conditions or medications.

Chapter 2

Coping With the Diagnosis

In This Chapter

- ◆ Coping with the news
- ◆ Moving through the stages of grief
- ◆ Telling friends and family
- ◆ Surfing the Internet

So you just got back from the doctor's office and your head is spinning. You have diabetes. What does that mean? How will it affect your life? How and when do you tell friends and family? And, most of all, what did you do to deserve this? You're likely scared, confused, and maybe even a little angry. That's fine. Those are all normal reactions to learning you have a chronic disease. Here's how to cope.

Take a Deep Breath

Literally. Take a deep breath. In, out. In, out. It's been nearly a century since a diagnosis of diabetes meant death. Today, it's a *chronic disease* that is inherently treatable. Depending on the severity of your disease, you might even be able to treat it with just some simple lifestyle changes and not even have to use any medication, at least for a while. In fact, the irony of this disease is that having been diagnosed with it, you can now begin to live a healthier lifestyle than you've ever before lived.

> **MedLingo**
>
> A **chronic disease** or disorder is one that doesn't go away with treatment. For instance, if you have strep throat, it can be cured with antibiotics. But a chronic condition such as diabetes cannot be cured; it can only be managed to enable you to live the fullest, healthiest life possible.

This Isn't Happening to Me

Forget denial. If you think the diagnosis was wrong, by all means seek a second opinion. You'll likely get the same results. Blood tests rarely lie. And no, that fantasy you've been having about the doctor's office mixing up your blood test with someone else's isn't going to come true.

"But I feel fine," you're thinking. "How could I possibly be sick?" Consider yourself lucky. Your doctor caught your diabetes before it got so bad that it began to make its presence known with symptoms like frequent urination, excessive thirst, and weight loss.

That means that the high blood sugar levels you've been walking around with aren't high enough to cause those symptoms. But don't be fooled. If they stay as high as they are for a long time, they *will* cause serious complications that can affect your eyes, kidneys, and the nerves in your legs.

Fortunately, there's still time to lower your blood sugar levels and delay (and maybe even prevent) those complications. But denying that you have a chronic condition called diabetes and refusing to seek treatment or change your lifestyle habits is a foolish, blind thing to do that will only result in one thing—you feeling sick.

Strangely Enough, I Feel Relieved

Actually, that's not so strange. After all, there are much worse things you could have been diagnosed with (terminal cancer, for one). And if you were one of the 25 percent of people with diabetes who experienced symptoms, you might have been imagining all sorts of terrible diagnoses.

Plus, now that you know what is wrong with you—and how to manage it—you can reclaim some of that sense of control you might have been feeling slip away from you.

This period of relief will probably be short-lived, however. Then you'll go on to experience some of the other emotions described here, beginning with anger.

But I'm So Darn Mad!

Yeah, we know. When you find out that you have a chronic illness, you often go through many of the same steps described in the groundbreaking work by Elisabeth Kübler Ross on death and dying. Denial, anger, bargaining, depression, and acceptance. So anger is to be expected.

You're probably angry that you might have to take medication every day, possibly even give yourself shots. You're angry that many of your favorite foods (particularly those decadent chocolate truffles) might be off limits now (or at least partially off limits). You're angry that the good health you took for granted, the ability to get through the day without thinking about things like blood glucose levels, diet, exercise, heart disease, eye disease, and so on, is now gone. Poof! Disappeared like a snowball in August.

That's okay. Get angry. Scream at your diabetes, tell it how much you hate it, how much you wish it would go away. But don't let the anger take you over. It takes a lot of energy to be angry, and you're going to need that energy to manage your disease in the coming months and years.

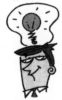

Sugar Sense

We all have a tendency to strike out at the people we love when we're angry or to engage in dangerous habits like overeating, drinking, or smoking—all of which can just make your diabetes worse. Instead, follow these tips to better cope with your anger without hurting anyone, including yourself:

- ◆ Write it down. Write a letter to your diabetes telling it how you feel now that it's moved into your life. Be honest. No one is going to see this letter except you.
- ◆ Draw a picture. Sometimes, we feel so angry that we don't know how to verbally express how we're feeling. So use a different part of your brain to draw a picture.
- ◆ Talk it out. Now might be the time to take a walk on a beach or in the woods with someone you love, where you can yell and scream and just be angry with your disease and trust that this person won't judge you.

Understand that this anger will probably always be with you in one form or another. For instance, you'll likely get angry or frustrated at some point with your treatment program—the restrictions on what you can eat, the constant need to exercise, the drugs you have to take. When that occurs, take a few minutes to feel and acknowledge that anger, and then remind yourself of the possible alternatives—blindness, kidney failure and dialysis, heart disease, strokes, amputations, and an earlier death—and continue on with the program that will stop these complications from occurring.

Let's Make a Deal

Ahh … you've entered the bargaining stage of grieving. You're saying to yourself, "If I _____ (eat better, lose weight, go for a walk every day, work less) maybe the diabetes will go away." You're thinking, well, I'll just find a better doctor. *He* (or she) will make me better.

Well, although doing those things can definitely improve your condition, it most often won't make diabetes go away. Losing enough weight if you're overweight or obese can make it disappear, but this is usually temporary. Unfortunately, you're forgetting the chronic nature of diabetes. To date, there is no cure and no way to make it go away entirely.

But I'm So Sad

It's quite common to become sad after you've been diagnosed with diabetes—or any chronic disease. You are grieving the loss of your old life, your old self. It's when that sadness begins interfering with your daily life that you need to be concerned. That's because people with diabetes might be more likely to be diagnosed with depression. In fact, several studies suggest that having diabetes doubles your risk of depression.

Depression is not something to take lightly. It is a dangerous disease that can sometimes be fatal. It is triggered by a variety of factors, including stress, medication, environmental factors, and difficult life events.

Also studies find that people with diabetes who are also depressed don't have very good control over their blood sugar levels and are more likely to have high levels of blood sugar. This in turn, can increase your risk of complications. The good news is this: treating depression leads to better control of your blood sugar levels, thus reducing your risk of complications.

Tipping the Balance into Depression

It is important that you be on the lookout for the symptoms of depression. Depression is a wily disease, sometimes camouflaging itself as anger or fatigue, sometimes sending you to sleep all the time, sometimes keeping you awake all night. It can come on as suddenly as a thunderstorm, or sneak up on you like night on a midsummer's day, gradually stealing your light until you find yourself sitting in darkness.

It is also a dangerous disease. In 2000, 29,350 people killed themselves in the United States. So, be alert for the following symptoms. If you experience five or more of them for more than two weeks, or have thoughts about hurting yourself, you should see your doctor immediately.

- Depressed mood on most days for most of each day

- Total or very noticeable loss of pleasure most of the time

- Significant increase or decrease in appetite, weight, or both

- Sleep disorders, either insomnia or excessive sleepiness, nearly every day

- Ongoing physical symptoms such as headaches or digestive disorders that don't respond to treatment

- Sexual dysfunction

- Feelings of agitation or a sense of intense slowness

- Loss of energy and a daily sense of tiredness

- Sense of guilt and worthlessness nearly all the time

- Excessive crying

- Inability to concentrate nearly every day

Having recurrent thoughts of death or suicide is a big red flag and you should definitely tell your doctor about it.

On Your Way to Feeling Better

The good news, however, is that depression is one of the most treatable diseases that doctors see. There's just one problem: less than half of

> **Sugar Sense** _____
>
> Worried about adding an antidepressant medication to your existing regimen of diabetes drugs? Don't be. Most prescription antidepressant medications are generally well tolerated and safe for people with diabetes.

all people suffering from depression nationwide receive adequate treatment, often because patients don't tell their doctors about their feelings.

You can't afford to be one of those people. Psychotherapy, medication, or a combination of both can make a huge difference in how you feel emotionally and physically. And that, in turn, will help you take better care of your diabetes. But you can't get started on your own. See your doctor.

Accepting the Reality

At some point, you should move into acceptance of your disease. There is no timeline for reaching this point; it could take weeks, or it might take years. Some people never accept their disease, refusing to move out of the denial or anger phase. Don't let that be you. The longer you wait to start treating your diabetes, the greater your chances will be of developing complications.

Reading this book is an excellent step to take on the road to acceptance. It shows you that many of your worst fears are groundless, that it is possible to live a full and healthy life with diabetes, and that you *can* regain some control over your health. The first step to control: tell the people in your life about your diagnosis.

Time to Tell

Hopefully, your partner or spouse was with you at the doctor's office when you first received your diagnosis so that he or she already knows about your diabetes. That still leaves an awful lot of other people to tell: your kids, your parents, other relatives, friends, co-workers. We discuss diabetes in the workplace in Chapter 15, but for now, let's focus on friends and family.

How to Tell

Here's what we *don't* recommend: "Hi, guys. I'm sick. I've got diabetes. Guess that means no more ice cream for me!" Instead, as with any serious news, you need to pick the right time and place to tell the people you care about and who care about you.

Find a quiet place where you won't be interrupted. Over dinner at a busy restaurant really isn't it. How about a quiet dinner at home? You can use the food you're eating as a good opening into discussing your condition.

It's also important that you think about what you want to say and how you want to say it. What is the message you want this person to receive? That you have a serious illness and are going to be sick? That you have a serious illness, but it's one that can be controlled? That you have a chronic condition that will mean some life changes, but most of them are actually good? You might try writing down some talking points, practicing in front of a mirror, or rehearsing with your spouse or partner.

Also remember that you're in control of the conversation. If the person you're talking with starts asking questions that make you feel uncomfortable, you can stop the conversation right there. Simply say, "I'd rather not discuss that right now." And, if you want the information about your condition to remain confidential, say so. Otherwise, you have no one to blame but yourself when the entire neighborhood learns about your disease and begins sending you sympathy cards.

Telling the Kids

How you tell your children that you have a chronic illness depends on the age of the child. If you have adult children, they have probably heard about diabetes and understand on some level what it means.

Don't be afraid to be completely honest with them about how serious your condition is and the kind of treatment plan you need to follow. Although you might want to continue thinking of them as children, they are adults. And because your disease likely has a genetic component to it, they now have a higher risk of developing diabetes. You have an opportunity to set an example in the right way to live with diabetes, so that if they are diagnosed with it one day, they won't have to go through the fear and anxiety you did.

If your children are little, then it's a good idea to dole out information in small chunks that they can understand. You might say something like, "Daddy has to make sure he doesn't get too much sugar from his food." Or "Mom has to watch what she eats so she doesn't get sick."

Keep in mind that your child may be frightened by your diagnosis. It is important to reassure her or him that you are not going to die and that with their help, they shouldn't see much, if any, change.

Warning

Make sure to keep all syringes, medications, and diabetes supplies out of reach of your children. If you have young children at home, always ask your pharmacist to put a child resistant cap on your medication.

One thing that might be particularly frightening to a child is seeing you giving yourself a shot of insulin, or even just testing your blood sugar with a glucose meter. After all, needles are scary to young kids. Calmly explain that this is how you get your medicine, and that it really doesn't hurt very much.

Telling Mom and Dad

Telling your parents might be a bit more complicated. Whether or not to tell them, and how to tell them, depends on your relationship with them and their own health.

Most people with diabetes are diagnosed in middle age, so your parents might be quite elderly. Can they comprehend the information you're giving them? Can they handle the shock of knowing that their child (for you will always be a child to them) has a chronic illness? Will they drive you bananas with worry, constantly calling to "see how you're doing?" If you answer yes to these questions, you might want to hold off on sharing the news.

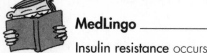

MedLingo

Insulin resistance occurs when your body is unable to respond to the insulin it produces.

But if you're close to one or both of your parents, see them frequently, and include them in your life in a major way, then you should probably tell them. Plus, as the disease is genetic in nature, it's quite likely your mom or dad has diabetes or *insulin resistance* (a kind of pre-diabetes). Sharing your experiences, creating new recipes, joining in an exercise program together, can make you all feel closer.

Telling Other Relatives

Who else you tell in your family is really up to you. After all, does cousin Johnny whom you haven't seen since your bar mitzvah really need to know? Certainly it's unlikely you need to make a concerted effort to reach all your long-lost aunts, uncles, and cousins and tell them about your condition.

But if there's a family event coming up—say, a wedding, communion, even a funeral—that might be a good time to mention it if the proper time arrives. For instance, if you're standing in the buffet line and your Uncle Pete asks why you're skipping the creamed corn, it might be a good time to casually mention that you have diabetes.

Telling Your Friends

You might be wondering why you even have to tell your friends about your diabetes. Well, maybe because they're your friends? If you trust and care about them, and they care about you, then you owe it to them to be honest.

Plus, if you spend any amount of time with them, they're going to notice that things are different. For instance, they might wonder why you're losing weight; why you no longer order a glass of wine before dinner; why you stopped lunching at All Things Fried and began dining at Super Salads.

There are numerous other reasons to tell your friends:

◆ They might have diabetes, too. No one understands what it's like to live with this disease better than someone who already has it.

◆ They can help you stick to your healthy eating plan when you're dining with them.

◆ They can serve as a walking or tennis partner to get you out there exercising. It's always easier to work out with a friend than alone.

◆ They can learn the signs of low blood sugar and serve as a warning system if you become hypoglycemic.

MedLingo

If you tell a friend about your diabetes and his or her response is negative (for instance, blaming it on your weight, becoming distant, or giving bad advice like telling you that one piece of cake won't hurt) then it's time to dump that "friend" and put your energy into finding a new one. Such "friends" can sabotage your efforts to remain healthy.

Is It My Fault?

You can barely pick up a newspaper today without reading about the "epidemic" of diabetes because Americans are too fat. And quite likely, you're also overweight. So it might be easy to think (or for others to think) that you caused this disease yourself by eating too much and exercising too little. Hold on. It's not quite that simple. If it were, then everyone who is overweight and a couch potato would have diabetes. Yes, definitely, being overweight and getting little physical activity can contribute to the development of diabetes. But some underlying genetic glitch lies at the heart of your disease; if it didn't exist, your body would find a way to compensate for the weight without flipping into full-blown diabetes.

Of course, knowing this might not prevent you from feeling ashamed of your diagnosis. And some days, you might feel as if you're walking around with a scarlet D around your neck—a mark of your weakness and shame. The Greeks had a name for this sense of shame: *stigma*. It can lead to social withdrawal, anxiety, and depression, all of which can make your diabetes worse.

So it is important to come to terms with the disease as simply that—a disease. Not as some punishment for the supersize lunches you've been eating or a retribution for the bag of chocolate kisses you inhaled last Christmas. Instead, help yourself move beyond those feelings of blame by doing your best to control your diabetes through a healthy lifestyle and good medical care.

> **Sugar Sense**
>
> Next time someone suggests that you developed diabetes because you ate too much, are too fat, don't exercise enough, and so on, tell the person that diabetes can happen to anyone—even thin people who follow a healthy diet.

Living With a Chronic Disease

You know that old saying: Today is the first day of the rest of your life? Well, it's really true when you've been diagnosed with diabetes. It's like a guest that just won't leave, so instead of constantly fighting it, you need to learn to live with it, build a guest room, clear a shelf in the refrigerator, set up some ground rules, etc.

One of the first things you should do is learn about your condition. You're making a good start with this book, but you should also spend some time out in cyberspace.

Time to Surf the Diabetes Web

Did you know that more people use the Internet to find health information than for just about any other purpose? (The other top reason people use the Internet is to look at pornography, but we're not going to go there!)

There's a reason for that; the Internet provides not only a mountain of information about your disease, but it's also a good meeting place to "talk" with others about diabetes, find doctors who specialize in the disease, keep up on the latest research, and even track your blood sugar levels. You can find recipes, virtual partners for exercising, newsletters, advice, and support.

Sorting the Wheat from the Chaff

If you type the word "diabetes" in the Google search engine and hit enter, you will wind up with over 35 million hits! It's enough to make you want to throw your computer through the window. That's one of the frustrating things about searching for information on the Internet; there's so much out there, and it's so hard to tell what's "good" information and what's not. Here are some tips to follow:

- ◆ Government websites (they end in .gov) generally have pretty reliable information.

- ◆ Websites from nonprofit organizations and associations (they end in .org), like the American Diabetes Association, also generally have pretty good information. However, keep in mind that anyone can register a site as a .org—it doesn't mean they're a nonprofit.

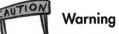

Warning _____

Never change your medication, diet, or exercise habits based simply on something you read on a website (or anywhere else). Always talk to your doctor first before changing anything in your treatment plan.

- ◆ Websites from academic medical centers (they end in .edu) also generally provide good, reliable information.

Always look to see who is sponsoring the website. If the sponsor is a drug company, for instance, the information provided might be biased toward getting you to try their product. Also check to see who reviewed the information and when it was last reviewed. Medical information changes so quickly that quality websites have all content reviewed on at least an annual basis, if not more frequently.

The following are some of the best, most reputable websites available for diabetes information. They're just starting points, though. Follow the links they provide ever deeper, and you'll soon find you have more than enough sites to explore. You'll find more sites in the Resources section at the back of this book.

- ◆ The American Diabetes Association
  www.diabetes.org

- ◆ The Centers for Disease Control's Division of Diabetes Translation
  www.cdc.gov/diabetes

- ◆ The National Diabetes Information Clearinghouse of the National Institutes of Health (NIH)
  http://diabetes.niddk.nih.gov

- The U.S. National Library of Medicine
  www.nlm.nih.gov/medlineplus/diabetes.html

- The U.S. Food and Drug Administration
  www.fda.gov/diabetes

- MEDLINE Plus
  www.nlm.nih.gov/medlineplus/diabetes.html

- David Mendosa's website
  www.mendosa.com

Sugar Sense

When surfing the Web for health information, the National Institutes of Health recommends you ask the following questions about websites:

- **Who runs this site?** The information should be clearly available.

- **Who pays for the site?** Even nonprofit organizations may accept pharmaceutical or other industry funding for their website.

- **What is the purpose of the site?** This should be clearly stated on the home page (or from a link from the home page).

- **Where does the information come from and what is the basis of the information?** The original source should be clearly labeled if it isn't original information. Look for references.

- **How is the information selected?** Is there an editorial board? Do the individuals running the site have professional and scientific qualifications? Is the information reviewed by a qualified individual?

- **How old is the information?** Things change quickly in medicine; quality healthcare sites should be reviewed at least once a year.

- **How does the website choose links to other sites?** Reliable websites usually have a policy regarding linkages.

- **What information is the website collecting about you?** If you have to register to use the website, beware; the owner is collecting information about you and you should ask why. Some sell this information to other marketers, some use it to market directly to you.

- **How does the website manage interactions with users?** Make sure there's a way for you to contact the website owners with questions or concerns.

Practice Safe Surfing

As you visit more sites about diabetes, you'll likely discover bulletin boards, listserves, and other online communities where you can "talk" with other people who have the disease about everything from what to serve for Christmas dinner to how to handle a vacation overseas.

These online communities are fabulous resources to find support and advice, and we encourage you to use them to your advantage. Just practice a few safe surfing rules:

- Never give out your full name, address, or phone number online.

- Set up a separate e-mail account from your primary e-mail account to use for these communications. This helps reduce the amount of spam, or junk e-mail, you receive to your primary e-mail address.

- Be wary of any "special offers," or anyone trying to sell you something to treat or help with your diabetes. Never give your credit card number or other personal financial information to anyone you don't know or trust.

Prepare for Bumps in the Road

Maybe you're feeling pretty good right about now. You've moved through the grief stages, you're learning to manage your disease through exercise, diet, and medication, and you've told the people in your life who matter most. They've been great—providing support and comfort just when you needed it most.

So it's smooth sailing from here on, right? Wrong. Remember that word, "chronic." Diabetes is a lifetime disease and nothing in our lives remains the same for very long. You're going to find over the coming months and years that you continually cycle back through the five stages of denial, anger, sadness, bargaining, and acceptance.

You'll have times of frustration when it seems you can't do anything right when it comes to controlling your blood sugar. Times of fear when your doctor tells you that she's noticed some blood vessel damage in your eyes. Times of depression when you feel left out during major holidays, which always seem to revolve around food.

The key to coping is not to deal with these issues as a whole, but to break them down and focus on them individually, one day at a time. For instance, instead of worrying about maintaining your blood sugar levels throughout the month or even a week, focus on maintaining them throughout the day. The weeks and months and years will take care of themselves.

The Least You Need to Know

- It is customary to go through various stages of grief, including anger and denial, after receiving a diagnosis of diabetes.

- People with diabetes have a high risk of being diagnosed with depression (and vice versa).

- Who, when, and how you tell your friends and family about your disease is up to you.

- The Internet provides an excellent place to find information about your disease.

Diabetes and Your Body

In This Chapter

- The importance of hormones
- A homeostatic system
- How the pancreas works
- How cells use insulin and glucose
- What goes wrong in type 2 diabetes

It's difficult to understand how diabetes develops and behaves in your body until you understand some of the *anatomy* and *physiology* involved in the disease, or how the organs involved work or don't work. Don't worry. We keep this simple and give you just as much as you need to know to understand the basics. After all, you're not going to medical school here, you're just trying to educate yourself about your disease!

It's a System, Silly

What's important to remember as you read through this chapter is that none of the parts we describe—whether the pancreas, liver, muscles, or hormones—exist on their own. They are all part of a whole, a system that, when it works right, exists in balance—not too much, not too little. This

MedLingo

Anatomy refers to the study of the parts and structure of the human body. **Physiology** refers to the study of how those parts function.

MedLingo

When the parts and their functions are all in balance, the body, or even certain systems in your body, is said to be in **homeostasis.**

MedLingo

The word **hormone** stems from a Greek word that means "to arouse," and hormones *arouse* cells to action.

balance is called *homeostasis*. When you fall out of homeostasis, problems like diabetes—or complications relating to diabetes—develop.

Another way to think about homeostasis is to picture an assembly line. The line is designed to move at a certain speed so that every part coming down the line can be carefully attached to the next part. If it begins moving too fast, the supervisor slows it down; if it's moving too slow, he or she speeds it up. As long as the line moves smoothly, everything works well and a car (or toy or can of beans) pops out at the end. But if one part of the line begins moving too fast without someone slowing it down, unfinished parts pile up at the other end.

Remember the scene in *I Love Lucy* when Lucy and Ethel were working in a candy factory and the conveyer belt began moving so fast they couldn't keep up? They started stuffing chocolates into their mouths as fast as possible, eventually making themselves sick. That's exactly what we *don't* want to happen to you.

An organ is made up of several tissues that have one or more specific functions. Some organs contain glands, which are structures that produce chemicals. If these chemicals leave the gland to work elsewhere in the body, they are called *hormones*.

Hormones, Hormones, Everywhere

The homeostasis that is so critical in diabetes is primarily controlled by the *endocrine system*, which coordinates and directs the activities of all your body's cells. It does this through the release of *hormones*, which are chemical messengers released into the blood by various *glands* throughout the body. The hormones travel to other parts of the body where they deliver specific instructions to organs or cells, called target organs or target cells.

Hormones control nearly every aspect of life: reproduction, growth and development, the immune system, the chemical balance of the blood, and the production of energy. It's this latter mechanism that we focus on.

Peering at the Pancreas

There are certain organs that, although important, we can really do quite nicely without. Consider the tonsils and the appendix. Not so with the pancreas. This astounding bit of news was discovered in 1879, when a German physician named Oscar Minkowski decided to remove a dog's pancreas. Suddenly, this dog began peeing in his cage, a previously unheard of action. When Minkowski tested the dog's urine, he found it filled with sugar. Voilà! He'd just become the first person to induce diabetes into another living thing.

That discovery—that the pancreas plays a role in diabetes—paved the way for most of what followed in our understanding of the disease.

> ![CAUTION] **Warning** _____
>
> Remaining in homeostasis or normal balance not only helps prevent disease, but is also crucial to managing your disease. If you fall out of homeostasis when you have diabetes (meaning that your blood sugars get too high or too low), you run into trouble. Blood sugar levels that remain too high increase your risk for complications. Too low, and you can't function normally. Additionally, if blood sugars are very high, you will suffer from the symptoms mentioned earlier, including increased urination, thirst, and possibly blurred vision. That's why U.K. Diabetes, the national diabetes organization for the United Kingdom, uses the hummingbird as its logo. It symbolizes the balance and control you must maintain when you have diabetes.

You Say Organ; I Say Gland

The pancreas, located close to the stomach in the abdominal cavity, is a pancake-like structure that lies across about two thirds the width of the abdomen. It is actually a gland. That means it produces hormones.

And although the pancreas does, indeed, play a critical role in the development of diabetes, regulating blood sugar is only part of its function. Its primary reason for being is to aid in digestion by producing enzymes that break down the food we eat into smaller units after it leaves the stomach so that it can enter the bloodstream. Because we're not too concerned about digestion in this book, we're going to skip over this part of the pancreas and focus on its role in diabetes. To do that, we have to visit a part of the pancreas called the islets of Langerhans, named after the researcher who first discovered them.

A Million Strong: The Islets of Langerhans

Technically, we no longer use the name, "Islets of Langerhans," although it does do a good job of describing what are now known as *pancreatic islets*. These are little masses of hormone-producing tissue scattered throughout the enzyme-producing parts of the pancreas. The islets make up only 1 percent of the pancreas.

These islets produce and release two hormones that work in opposite directions: insulin and *glucagon*. Insulin is made, stored, and eventually released by special cells within the pancreatic islets called *beta cells*. Glucagon is made, stored, and released by the *alpha cells* of the pancreatic islets. They work against each other, but together they help keep your blood sugar levels normal.

A Sugar by Any Other Name: Glucose

What happens when you run out of gas for your car? The car stops, right? The same thing happens if your blood sugar levels get too low. You get dizzy, have trouble thinking straight, feel shaky, start to sweat, and feel your heart pounding in your chest. If your blood sugar gets too low, you might even pass out.

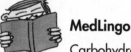

MedLingo

Carbohydrates are organic compounds composed of carbon, oxygen and hydrogen. Starches, sugars and cellulose are carbohydrates.

That's the importance of glucose, a.k.a. "blood sugar." Every time you eat, the food you take in is broken down into simpler elements that your cells can use, and one of the most basic is glucose—a simple *carbohydrate*.

The Unbroken Circle: Regulating Blood Sugar

Although some parts of the body can store glucose in various forms for later use, the brain and other parts of the nervous system need a constant, regular supply. One way to get that is to eat carbohydrates all the time.

Of course, that's not practical, and besides, you'd weigh almost 500 pounds. So the body has developed a complex feedback system to maintain a steady supply of glucose to the brain and other organs.

Bet You Didn't Know

How many famous people can you name who have type 2 diabetes? How about actresses Delta Burke and Halle Berry, boxer Sugar Ray Robinson, baseball star Jackie Robinson, and novelist H. G. Wells, just to mention a few. Good to know you're in good company, right?

After Eating

About 10 minutes after you start eating a meal, your digestive system begins breaking down the food into smaller nutrients for your body to use, including glucose from carbohydrates. These nutrients then enter your bloodstream.

So now you have all this glucose floating around in your blood (actually, only about a teaspoon at any one time if you're healthy). It's not doing much good in your blood; it has to get *into* your cells.

Getting Glucose into Cells

Glucose gets into certain tissues (the brain, other parts of the nervous system, liver, red blood cells, and kidney cells) that require it for energy by attaching to certain "buckets" called *glucose transporters*. These "buckets" lie on the outside of the cell *membrane*. They act like ferry boats, carrying the glucose into the inner workings of the cell where it can be transformed into energy.

Most of the rest of the glucose in your blood gets stored in muscle and liver, with a bit saved up in fat tissue. In muscle and fat tissues, the glucose transporters start out *inside* the cell, not on the outside membrane. Their challenge is to get to the cell's outside membrane so that they can pick up the glucose and carry it into the cells. In the liver, the glucose transporters are already on the outside membrane.

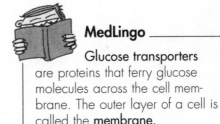

MedLingo

Glucose transporters are proteins that ferry glucose molecules across the cell membrane. The outer layer of a cell is called the **membrane**.

Insulin to the Rescue!

The key to keeping blood glucose levels normal is insulin. Through a complex system of signals, your pancreas gets word that your digestive system is processing food and that there's a bunch of glucose hanging out in your blood. The signals get transferred to your beta cells, which begin putting out insulin.

> **MedLingo** _____
> Receptors are special proteins within or on the outside of cells designed to bind to certain chemicals within the body.

The insulin heads out into the bloodstream looking for muscle, liver, and adipose tissue, or fat cells. When insulin reaches these tissues, it latches onto special _receptors_ on these cells, called insulin receptors, to create a kind of lock-and-key mechanism. The receptors are the lock; insulin is the key. What happens next depends on which tissue the insulin attaches.

In the liver, insulin keeps this organ from producing glucose at the same time that glucose is entering the bloodstream from the food we just ate. We discuss this more later.

When insulin attaches itself to the receptors on muscle and fat, the glucose transporters within the cells are free to move to the outside membrane. There, these little ferry boats act like they do on other tissues—carrying glucose molecules through the cell membrane into the inner workings of the cell itself.

What to Do with the Extra

When glucose enters any cell, it is used for energy to keep that cell working. Extra glucose not needed for energy is stored as another form of carbohydrate called _glycogen_ (not to be confused with glucagon).

> **MedLingo** _____
> In most cells, many glucose molecules attach themselves together and are stored as **glycogen**. When glycogen changes back into **glucose**, the glucose can be used for energy.

Because muscle and liver tissue can also use another type of fuel called fatty acids for energy, these tissues don't need a lot of glucose for energy. Thus, they store much of the glucose they get as _glycogen_.

Extra glucose entering fat cells is changed to, well, fat. Keep this in mind; it will be important later on when we talk about the connection between weight and diabetes.

What About Between Meals?

In between meals, when food doesn't supply the glucose, it's up to the liver to produce enough to keep your brain working. This is the only time the liver produces glucose, because if you were getting sugar from both it *and* your food, your blood sugar levels would be too high.

The liver gets word about whether or not it should produce glucose or not through a lovely little feedback loop that works like this: as blood glucose begins to rise above normal, beta cells produce a little extra insulin that goes to the liver and tells the liver to slow its production of glucose.

As soon as blood glucose begins to drop below normal, the beta cells stop producing insulin and alpha cells in the pancreas (remember them?) release glucagon. This glucagon also heads right to the liver and tells it to produce a little *extra* glucose.

In this way, there is a minute-to-minute regulation between insulin and glucagon, which work on the liver in opposite directions, to keep blood sugar levels normal between meals and, more important, overnight when you're not eating.

So What's Going On in Fat Tissue?

Glucagon has a somewhat different effect on adipose tissue cells (a.k.a. fat), where it stimulates cells to break down the stored fat (called triglycerides) to fatty acids and a form of sugar called *glycerol*.

And where do the glycerol and fatty acids go? One place is to the liver! There, the glycerol is turned back into glucose. In addition, fatty acids stimulate the metabolic machinery that combines the glycerol with other building blocks for glucose (like amino acids that come from the breakdown of proteins) into glucose.

MedLingo

Glycerol is a form of sugar (one half of a glucose molecule) produced when fat cells break down triglycerides.

This, in turn, helps raise blood sugar levels, which stimulates the release of insulin, which starts the whole process all over again. In this way, you have a continuous source of energy without having to continually eat. You can see how this works in the following illustration of the feedback loop between glucagon and insulin.

Falling Out of Normal Balance: Diabetes

Okay, so now you know how things *should* work. Now here's what's going on in *your* body.

In type 2 diabetes, your body is still producing insulin—probably a fair amount of insulin, particularly if you're overweight or obese. It's just not producing enough to keep your blood sugar levels normal. If you're thin and have type 2 diabetes, it's likely that your body isn't producing enough insulin to begin with.

The problem is that your body doesn't respond to this insulin normally. In other words, the insulin is not having the desired effect on your muscle cells. They, in turn, aren't moving those little glucose transporters from inside the cell to the membrane on the outside of the cell. And that means that glucose builds up in your blood.

Much of what determines how well insulin works in our body is inherited from our parents, but we don't know *how* it is inherited. We do know that if insulin isn't working well in your body, then you have a condition called *insulin resistance*. Even if you have insulin resistance, as long as your beta cells can put out enough insulin to overcome the resistance, you won't get diabetes. Nonethe-less, you're still left with blood insulin levels that are higher than normal, a condition called *hyperinsulinemia*, which can be dangerous in and of itself.

Plus, if the beta cells can't keep up with the extra demand placed on them, they start to poop out and you get type 2 diabetes. We don't know why the beta cells run out of steam only in some people with insulin resistance while not in others, but this, too, seems to be inherited.

Whatever the reason, there's not enough insulin to get glucose into muscle and fat cells. Also there's not enough insulin to tell your liver to *stop* making glucose. Thus, your blood glucose levels get too high and you're in trouble.

MedLingo

Hyperinsulinemia occurs when you have increased levels of insulin in your blood because your pancreatic beta cells are producing too much insulin. In some cases, this occurs because your liver isn't doing a good enough job of removing excess insulin.

Insulin resistance occurs when your body can't use the insulin your pancreas produces.

Bet You Didn't Know

Ever wonder why your blood glucose levels are always so high in the morning even before you've eaten breakfast? Easy: As your beta cells continue to poop out, producing less and less insulin, they don't send enough insulin to your liver to tell it to stop producing glucose. So your liver is pumping out glucose all night, regardless of how high your blood levels get, because there's not enough insulin coming in to turn off the production. Now you eat breakfast, sending even *more* glucose into your bloodstream and sending your blood sugar levels even higher. Result? You guessed it: Trouble.

Behind the Symptoms of Diabetes

Now that you understand how the system works (and what happens when it's not working), let's look at the reason for the symptoms you can get if your blood glucose levels get too high. If you have any of these, pay attention. Your body is trying to tell you something.

- **Thirst and excessive urination.** One of the first clues that blood glucose is too high is that you have to pee all the time. This occurs because blood normally cycles through your kidneys, which removes wastes for, uh, disposal. At the same time, the kidneys normally return glucose that goes through them back into the bloodstream. But if you have large amounts of glucose in your blood, your kidneys can't handle it all. The excess "spills" over into urine. All that excess sugar draws in water like how dry rice absorbs liquid when it's being cooked. That extra water goes into the urine, and the result is that you pee more (excess urination). This leads to dehydration (not enough fluid in the blood stream), prompting you to drink more, in other words, increased thirst, which leads to more urination, and so on and so on.

- **Fatigue.** This is a simple one. If your cells aren't getting the energy they need from glucose, they can't produce energy, ergo a walk around the block can leave you feeling as wiped out as if you'd just run a 5K marathon.

- **Blurred vision.** If blood sugar levels are too high, sugar builds up in your eyes. This excess sugar also draws in fluid, changing the shape of the lens in your eye and making your vision blurry.

- **Increased hunger and weight loss.** Again, an easy one. If your cells aren't getting enough glucose for energy, signals go out for your body to bring in more glucose, i.e., eat more. Yet because the glucose from food can't be used for energy very well, your body also sends out signals to break down stored fat for energy, and you lose weight.

Bet You Didn't Know

Although no one knows for sure what causes type 2 diabetes, several theories are under investigation:

♦ Something is wrong with your beta cells. Early in the disease, they don't release insulin fast enough after you eat, so the blood levels of glucose (from your food) get too high. Later on in the disease, as the beta cells get weaker, not enough insulin is produced.

♦ You don't have enough beta cells.

♦ You inherited some genetic mutation from one or both of your parents that wreaks havoc with the feedback system regulating blood sugar levels. There definitely is some kind of genetic reason. Just consider that simply because you have type 2 diabetes, your children have a 25 to 30 percent chance of developing the disease, especially if they are overweight or obese. If both their parents have it, they have a 50 to 75 percent chance.

The Least You Need to Know

♦ If your body doesn't stay in normal balance, or homeostasis, illnesses like diabetes tend to occur.

♦ Most patients with type 2 diabetes have insulin resistance, which develops when beta cells can't keep up with the extra demand placed upon them as a result of insulin resistance.

♦ The pancreas is the gland/organ that plays a large role in diabetes. It produces two important hormones: insulin, released when blood sugar levels are high, and glucagon, released when blood sugar levels are low.

♦ Insulin is required to get glucose into muscle and fat cells and to get the liver to stop producing glucose right after we eat.

♦ Insulin is also important because it tells the liver to produce just enough glucose between meals and overnight to keep our blood sugars normal.

Part 2

Traveling the Treatment Trail

This section of the book helps you choose the team of healthcare professionals who will treat you—from your doctor to your nutritionist to your diabetes educator. In Chapters 5 and 6, you'll learn about the key lifestyle changes you'll need to make to manage your diabetes and blood sugar levels, namely, exercise and diet. The next two chapters address medical treatment of diabetes—from pills to insulin, while Chapter 9 explores the growing use of insulin pumps among people with type 2 diabetes. And in Chapter 10, we tell you a bit about alternative therapies that might provide additional benefits with your regular treatment—and those that won't.

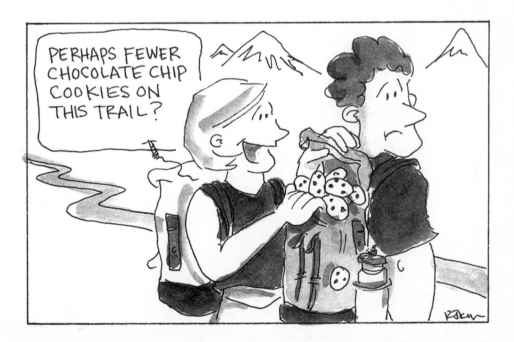

Chapter 4

Assembling Your Treatment Team

In This Chapter

- Finding the right members of your medical team
- Anticipating the costs
- Handling the insurance side of things
- What to do if you're uninsured

You probably already have a doctor; most likely, he or she diagnosed your diabetes. But the doctor you've been seeing for strep throat, a sore back, and annual checkups may not be the only doctor you need anymore.

Not only that, but you will probably need to bring in other medical professionals—ranging from nurses to nutritionists—to help you manage your diabetes. This is your treatment team, and they're a vital part of your diabetes treatment program.

What's Up, Doc? Finding the Right Doctor

If you're like most people, you receive the majority of your medical care from a primary care physician—typically either an internal medicine specialist or a family practitioner. And there's no reason to stop. The majority of people with diabetes are treated by primary care physicians, and diabetes is the seventh most common reason for a visit to a primary care physician. But which primary care physician is right for you?

Just as any other physician, both family practitioners and internists spend four years in medical school and then three more years in *residency* training. Internists spend all of their time learning about diseases in adults while family practitioners are more broadly trained in pediatrics, orthopedics and obstetrics/gynecology as well as diseases in adults. Thus, internists receive more training in treating people with diabetes.

MedLingo

Before they can be licensed to practice medicine, physicians must complete a **residency,** which is several years of training in a hospital setting under the guidance of more experienced physicians.

When they hang out their shingle, they share some similarities. For instance, each is trained to treat a wide variety of general medical conditions. But there are some differences between the two.

Warning

Make sure your doctor is board-certified in his or her specialty. Board certified means that the doctor has completed the necessary training and passed a special examination to become certified by a member of the American Board of Medical Specialties (ABMS), an organization of 24 approved medical specialty boards. Furthermore, to keep their board certification, doctors must take and pass a test every few years.

Internal medicine specialists are board certified by the American Board of Internal Medicine. They may also be board certified in a subspecialty, such as cardiology or endocrinology, diabetes, and metabolism after taking two or more years of additional training (called a fellowship) in these areas. Family practitioners are board certified by the American Board of Family Medicine.

Most hospitals and insurance companies require that physicians be board certified to practice at the hospital or to see patients as part of a Health Maintenance Organization (HMO).

Fun with Your Family Practitioner

Family practitioners do just what their name implies: treat the whole family. They are trained to provide care to adults as well as children. In some rural areas, family practitioners might serve as a kind of doctor-of-all, even performing some minor surgeries and delivering babies. But in most areas of the country, they tend to handle the more routine patient care, referring patients to specialists for more complex care.

Of Internists, Family Practitioners, and Diabetes

Although what we're about to say here might make some primary care doctors mad (sorry!), the fact is, if you have diabetes, you're probably better off choosing a doctor who has a lot of experience taking care of people with diabetes as your primary care physician. In some cases, that might be an internist.

In general, internal medicine doctors tend to treat older patients (they don't see children), who are more likely to have diabetes. It's a well-known fact in medicine (as in anything in life, actually) that the more you do something, the better you get at it. So the more diabetes patients an internist (or a family practitioner) treats, the better he or she will be at managing the condition and its complications. Some internists, and even a few family practitioners, turn their entire practices over to patients with diabetes.

> **MedLingo**
> _Endocrinology_ is a special field of medicine devoted to dealing with disorders of the endocrine system and hormonal disorders, including diabetes.

Plus, some internists have special training in the field of *endocrinology*. Some are even board-certified in endocrinology, meaning that they have completed a fellowship (additional training) in the field and passed a certification test in endocrinology.

Was It Something I Said?

Even if you feel comfortable with the care your primary care doctor provides, chances are that you may be referred to a specialist at one point or another. Don't take this personally! Your doctor is not trying to get rid of you. Rather, he or she is trying to ensure that you get the best care possible. That sometimes means seeing a doctor with additional training in certain areas.

When you are referred to another doctor, your primary care doctor still remains involved in your care. The referring doctor should be sending your primary care doctor regular reports on your care and, in many instances, will send you "back" to your family doctor after your condition is under control. So, for instance, you might see an endocrinologist (more on that later) for your diabetes once every three months; but you'll still see your family doctor for routine care, even of your diabetes, throughout the year.

Bet You Didn't Know

The specialists you might see for your diabetes and associated complications could include these:

◆ **Cardiologist:** focused on the care of your heart.

◆ **Nephrologist:** focused on the care of your kidneys.

◆ **Ophthalmologist:** focused on the care of your eyes.

◆ **Vascular surgeon:** focused on care of the blood vessels in your legs.

Finding the Right Doc: Asking Around

Close those Yellow Pages and step away from the book. Now! That's no way to find a good doctor. The best way is to begin asking around. Ask friends, neighbors, relatives, even the guy who delivers your newspaper. Who is their primary care doctor, and why do they like him or her?

That's only a place to start, however. You also want to make sure that you find a doctor who is able to take care of your diabetes well. If you're new to an area, you can check with local hospitals. They often have referral lines that can match your particular needs with a suitable physician. You can also ask other health professionals such as your dentist, pharmacist, or even chiropractor for recommendations. When you have several names, it's time to check them out. Before you do, however, it's important to realize that your insurance plan will only cover your care if the doctors you see have a contract with them. If you see a doctor outside of your plan, you will usually have to pay more.

Interviewing Your Doctor

When you have diabetes, you can plan on seeing your doctor pretty often—at least once every three months when your condition is stable, or more frequently if it's not.

So you want to pick a doctor you like, feel comfortable with, can communicate with, and enjoy visiting (well, as much as anyone can enjoy seeing a doctor).

This is more important than you might think. Studies find that the more satisfied you are with your physician and the better the relationship is between the two of you, the more likely you are to follow your treatment plan. One study even found that patients who were unhappy with the patient/doctor relationship had higher blood sugar levels over time.

So it might be worth the money to make an appointment simply to meet the doctor and interview him or her. You will probably have to pay for this yourself, because most insurance companies won't cover it and few doctors today can afford to give up even 10 minutes of their time for free.

During the appointment, tell your doctor about yourself and your condition. Also talk about the kind of relationship you're looking for. Do you want a doctor who supports the use of alternative therapies as well as traditional therapies? Someone who is quick to refer you to other specialists? Someone who will follow you if you are hospitalized? These are all issues you need to discuss.

What About the Office?

No matter how great your doctor is, if the office is an unorganized mess, it will make your life miserable. So check out how the office runs. Here are some things to consider:

◆ How long is the typical wait for a nonemergency appointment? What if there is an emergency?

◆ How long did you have to wait before you saw the doctor?

◆ How organized does the office seem? Were they able to find your paperwork and quickly make a copy of your health-insurance card?

◆ Do they accept your health insurance? Will they file all the paperwork for you or do you have to do it?

◆ Is the office conveniently located, or does the doctor have multiple locations (and may be far away on a day you need to be seen)?

◆ Will you always see *your* doctor, or will you see other doctors in the practice?

The Real Question: Primary Care Doctor or Endocrinologist?

So, you're thinking, if my doctor is just going to refer me to an endocrinologist anyway, why not just go to one all the time as my primary care doctor? Good question.

Studies do find that people with diabetes who have their care coordinated by an endocrinologist generally do better overall than those whose care is coordinated by a primary care doctor. And that makes sense when you figure that endocrinologists probably treat a lot more patients with diabetes than most primary care doctors do.

But there are far fewer endocrinologists in the country than there are primary care doctors (about 3,000 that see people with diabetes compared to more than 94,000 family practitioners and 177,000 internists), meaning that they're not very accessible, especially if you live in a rural area.

Plus, because they're specialists, their care usually costs more. And if you get sick with something unrelated to your diabetes, like the flu or allergies, you still have to see your primary care physician in most cases. Some endocrinologists will, however, also take on the primary care of their patients. If you can find one who does (and meets your other requirements), you might consider signing on with that individual for all of your health care.

Because those kind of endocrinologists are few and far between, you're probably better off seeing one soon after your diagnosis, and then periodically thereafter, but continuing to leave the bulk of your medical management (a fancy word for healthcare) up to your regular doctor.

Why Do I Need a Diabetes Educator?

As you probably already know, treating diabetes is much more complicated than simply writing a prescription for insulin and checking your blood sugar. So much of diabetes care revolves around lifestyle management such as diet, exercise, and careful tracking of your blood sugar levels. This requires a lot of explaining and education that today's doctors simply do not have time for.

Thank goodness, then, for diabetes educators. Diabetes educators are specially trained and certified health professionals who provide information to help you live a healthier life with diabetes. They can be nurses, dietitians, pharmacists, social workers, exercise physiologists, or even doctors.

Bet You Didn't Know

To become a certified diabetes educator, a dietitian (or any other professional for that matter) must have a minimum of two years of professional practice experience in diabetes self-management training, and at least 1,000 hours of hands-on experience in diabetes self-management with patients. They must be currently employed as a diabetes educator for at least four hours a week and they must pass a tough written examination.

Although some diabetes educators work in doctors' offices, many work in the community, often holding classes for local hospitals, large medical groups, and community clinics. Some work in nursing homes, where large numbers of residents with diabetes are likely to live.

Finding a diabetes educator in your area is easy. Just visit the American Association of Diabetes Educators online at www.aade.org, or call the Association (see Appendix A) to find an educator near you.

What Do They Do?

Diabetes educators can do everything from explaining what diabetes is and how it can affect you to helping design a personalized diet plan for you and mapping out a good walking route in your town. They teach you not only how to give yourself insulin if that's required, but also how to test your blood sugar levels and track the results.

They're often just a phone call or e-mail away if you have questions, and are usually far easier to reach with routine questions than your doctor.

Bet You Didn't Know

Some communities are experimenting with diabetes education telemedicine, in which diabetes educators "talk" to you over the phone or computer. Studies find that this works just as well at helping you to manage your condition and to reduce the stress related to diabetes as meeting with a diabetes educator in person.

Studies also find that the kind of diabetes self-management that diabetes educators teach can help improve your blood sugar control, your own care of yourself, your emotional well-being, and can lower the overall cost of your medical care.

Unfortunately, many insurance plans do not cover diabetes education, so you might need to pay for these services out of your own pocket.

Do I Need a Dietitian (Nutritionist)?

It depends. If your diabetes educator can also function as a nutritionist, that's great. But because diet is such a major part of any treatment plan for diabetes, a nutritionist is an important part of your team. Ideally, look for a certified diabetes educator who is also a registered dietitian (many are). You can find a registered dietitian at the American Dietetic Association's website at www.eatright.org.

Sugar Sense

Working with a nutritionist to receive medical nutrition therapy can not only improve your blood sugar control, but can also save you money because you might be able to use less medication.

Sugar Sense

It's quite likely that you'll learn some surprising information in your visits with your dietitian; for instance, you'll learn that avoiding sugar in your diet isn't the best way to control your blood sugar.

The dietitian (whom we'll call "she" for ease of writing) will help you complete a food diary to track what you've been eating so that she can determine how your diet needs to change. She will also help you to understand the signs and proper treatment of hyperglycemia, how your medications work in relationship to your food, and how exercise and eating play off one another.

She can also help you plan special menus for special events, adjust your diet when you're ill or under a great deal of stress, and recommend places to buy healthy foods that work well for people with diabetes. She'll even teach you how to read food labels (not as easy as you might think!) and how to order healthy foods in restaurants. So yes, in the end, we would definitely say that you *do* need a nutritionist who specializes in diabetes.

Again, however, many insurance plans do not cover the services of dietitians, so you might find yourself footing the bill on your own. Trust us; it's a worthwhile investment.

The Team Approach

The name of this chapter is "Assembling Your Treatment Team," and that's just how you have to look at your diabetes care. You have put together this important team—which might also include a social worker (to help with insurance information, recommend community resources, and help with some short-term therapy if you need someone to talk to), but you can't forget the most important member of the team: You!

No matter how good the members of your team are, they can't do a very good job if you do not share information with them (and follow their advice!). Specifically, you need to make sure that the members of your team know about the following:

◆ All drugs (prescription, over-the-counter, and even illegal) you're taking. If another doctor prescribes something new for you, make sure the healthcare provider who manages most of your diabetes care knows about it.

◆ Any herbs, vitamins, minerals, or other supplements you're taking.

◆ Any unusual stress you're under.

◆ How much alcohol you drink (be honest, now!).

◆ Your blood glucose values measured at home, when you measured them (dates and times, especially in relation to meals) and if anything out of the ordinary happened that might have influenced any of the individual values.

Sugar Sense _____

Carry a small notebook with you at all times that lists the brand name and dosage of your medication(s). Update it frequently. In case of an emergency, you'll have it with you.

Looking Out for Number One

You might think that it's up to your doctor to know what to check for during every visit and what to ask you. Well, that poor doctor probably has to see another 40 patients that day—so you can understand why he or she might be feeling slightly overwhelmed and even a little scattered. So take some time to reintroduce yourself when the doctor comes in and provide a brief (very brief) medical history, focused on any changes since the last time you saw your doctor.

If you think that your blood sugar levels are not under good-enough control (based on what you learn in later chapters), then make sure you bring it up with your doctor. You have to be your own best advocate, so complain (nicely!) when things aren't working.

Warning _____

If you're taking insulin, the American Diabetes Association recommends that you see your doctor at least four times a year. Otherwise, the association recommends two to four times a year if there are no problems or complications.

Also make sure someone weighs you and takes your blood and blood pressure while you're in the office and tests your blood for sugar levels, cholesterol levels, and any other needed tests.

Other things your doctor should ask about:

♦ How often you've had high or low blood glucose levels since your last visit

♦ Any changes you've made in your treatment program

♦ Any problems you're having following your program

♦ Any symptoms or health problems you've noticed

The doctor should also do the following:

♦ Review your blood glucose records.

♦ Check your feet. This is very important because most amputations of the toes, feet, and legs in this country occur in people with diabetes. Almost all could be avoided if the early signs of danger were picked up and treated.

♦ Take blood for an *HgA1c measurement.*

♦ Take a urine sample every year to check for protein.

♦ Refer you to an eye doctor (ophthalmologist) or to an optometrist who knows about diabetic eye disease for a dilated eye examination. We talk more about the importance of eye exams in Chapter 18.

MedLingo

An HgA1c, also known as a glycated hemoglobin measurement, hemoglobin A1c, or simply as an A1c, is a blood test that provides a picture of your blood glucose levels for the past three or four months. Therefore, high levels indicate that you've had problems controlling your blood sugar for a long time before the test.

When you visit your doctor, there are numerous tests and examinations you should receive and several important goals you need to meet in your diabetes management to avoid complications. We discuss these throughout this book.

Your doctor knows what these tests and goals are. But because today's physicians are so busy, and because you might be feeling fine and not think you need these tests, doctors often don't think to order the tests, which means you may not meet your treatment goals.

So in a way, you need to be your own doctor to make sure that this doesn't happen. The health record card in the following figure will help. It lists all the tests and examinations you need, when you need them, and what goals you should be aiming for.

Diabetes Health Record

Discuss these *Basic Guidelines for Diabetes Care* with your diabetes care provider and use this to record your results. Fold to fit into your wallet.

Take charge of your diabetes!

Review Blood Sugar Records (every visit) Target (pre-meals):	Date:			
Blood Pressure (every visit) Target:	Date:			
	Value:			
Weight (every visit) Target:	Date:			
	Value:			
Foot Exam (every visit)	Date:			
A1C Blood test to measure past 3 mos. blood sugar level (every 3 months) Target:	Date:			
	Value:			
Microalbuminuria Urine kidney test (every year) Target:	Date:			
	Value:			
Dilated Eye Exam (every year)	Date:			
Blood tests to measure "fats" important to heart disease				
Cholesterol (every visit) Target:	Date:			
	Value:			
Triglycerides (every year) Target:	Date:			
	Value:			
HDL / LDL (every year) Target:	Date:			
	Value:			
Flu Shots (every year)	Date:			
Pneumonia Vaccine (at least once/ask Dr.)				
Other				

Discuss these issues regularly with your health care provider to improve your diabetes management skills:

- Smoking Counseling
- Medications
- Nutrition Therapy
- Physical Activity
- Weight Management
- Complications
- Aspirin Therapy
- Hypoglycemia (low sugar)
- Hyperglycemia (high sugar)
- Sick Day Rules
- Psychosocial Issues
- Pre-pregnancy Counseling
- Pregnancy Management
- Dental Exams, twice yearly

Note: You may require other tests that are not listed.

Diabetes Health Record

_____
Your Name

_____
Diabetes Care Provider

_____
Diabetes Care Provider Telephone

_____
Medical Record Number

All people with diabetes need to learn diabetes self-care skills.

Take Charge of Your Diabetes!

All people with diabetes need to be actively involved in managing their diabetes. Do you know what tests you need to take care of your health and help you manage your diabetes? The *Diabetes Health Record* will help you keep track of the basic tests you need and how often you need them. It will also help you to record and remember the results of these tests.

The Diabetes Health Record is based on the *Basic Guidelines for Diabetes Care* developed by the Diabetes Coalition of California, in collaboration with the California Diabetes Prevention and Control Program, American Diabetes Association, and the Juvenile Diabetes Research Foundation International.

Juvenile Diabetes Research Foundation International

To order the **Basic Guidelines for Diabetes Care, Diabetes Health Record** and the ***Take Charge!*** training tool, call (916) 552-9888 or check www.caldiabetes.org

Diabetes Health Record Card

Make a copy of this card and keep it in your wallet so that you have it with you whenever you visit your doctor. Make sure your doctor does everything suggested on this card during your visit, and ask him or her to write your results on the back after each visit so that you can track your progress. The card is available in 14 different languages and can be downloaded from www.caldiabetes.org.

Paying for It All: Navigating the Labyrinth of Insurance

It ain't cheap having diabetes. Various estimates pin the cost at between $10,000 and $14,000 a year for medical expenses, compared to about $2,560 if you don't have diabetes. So having adequate health insurance coverage when you have diabetes is no small thing. Studies find that people whose insurance covers such things as testing supplies and medications have better overall control of their blood sugar than those who are uninsured or whose insurance plans don't cover such items.

If you're like many Americans under age 65, you probably get your health insurance from your employer (about two thirds of us do). And like most such individuals, you're probably paying more each year for the privilege. Keep paying it. As long as you were insured at the time of your diagnosis and you are part of an employer plan, your health insurance company cannot cancel or otherwise change your policy.

The Alphabet Soup of Managed Care

If you have employer-provided health insurance or even pay for your policy on your own, you likely have some form of a managed care plan. Maybe it's an HMO (a health maintenance plan), a PPO (a preferred provider plan), or a POS (a point-of-service option). The differences between these three plans used to be fairly significant in the early days of the managed care boom (the 1980s through the mid-90s). Today, there's not as much difference.

MedLingo

Most managed care plans contract with a group of physicians who agree to provide care for a certain reimbursement. This is called the **network**.

Basically, managed care plans try to "manage" costs as well as your care by restricting your care to a certain *network* of providers (physicians, hospitals, physical therapists, and so on) with whom the plan has negotiated a fixed payment. Some plans require that you get a referral from your primary care physician before seeing any specialist, such as an endocrinologist. Others simply make you pay more if you see a specialist or other doctor who isn't on the "approved" list.

Managed care plans have gotten a lot of bad press over the years, which is one reason they have become much less restrictive. Not all the bad press was deserved; in some areas, such as diabetes care, for instance, some managed care plans have done a really great job. They do this by implementing disease management programs, which is a comprehensive approach to diabetes care discussed in more detail later in this chapter.

Harkening Back to the Past: The Return of the Indemnity Plan

In the early days of health insurance, most plans were *indemnity* plans. They went out of favor during the managed care boom, but have been slowly creeping back.

In an indemnity plan (also called fee-for-service plan), you pay for medical services as you use them. Typically, you (or your employer) pay for the plan through *premiums*, and the plan pays for most of your medical care—after you've met a *deductible*. Most plans also require that you pay a *co-insurance* amount, typically a percentage of the approved reimbursement, usually between 20 and 30 percent.

The deductible can range from as little as $200 a year to as much as thousands of dollars. The beauty of the indemnity plan is that no one questions who you see or why you see a doctor. As long as your visit is covered under your plan's benefits, it is paid. Also, the cost of the plan is often tied to the amount of care used by an entire group of employees.

> **MedLingo**
>
> An **indemnity plan** is one in which medical services are paid for as they are used. A **premium** is the amount you pay each month or each year for a health insurance policy. Often, your employer pays part and you pay part. A **deductible** is the annual amount you must pay toward your health insurance costs before your health insurance company begins paying for services. **Co-insurance** is the percentage of a medical fee you must pay; your insurance plan pays the rest.

As health insurance costs have risen in recent years, these plans have come back into vogue. They're great in terms of freedom—you can see any doctor, any time, and go to any hospital. But they will probably cost you more. So compare costs carefully when you're deciding between an indemnity and a managed care plan. What's more important to you: freedom of choice or cost?

Aaack! I Lost My Job!

All bets are off if you lose your job or your employer decides to no longer offer healthcare coverage. That's why it's important to know your health insurance rights:

◆ COBRA: No, it's not a snake. COBRA stands for the Consolidated Omnibus Budget Reconciliation Act. This 1986 law allows you and your dependents to continue on your employer's insurance plan for another 18 to 36 months as long as you pay the entire premium (the amount you were paying plus the amount the employer was paying on your behalf). Generally, the employer must have 20 or more workers for you to be covered under COBRA.

◆ HIPAA: More alphabet soup, yes, but more protection. This is the Health Insurance Portability and Accountability Act of 1996. Among other things, it requires that if you lose your group health coverage (such as through your employer) you are guaranteed an offer of at least two health insurance policies that do not have any *pre-existing condition* exclusion periods. You have to meet certain criteria, however. For instance, you can't be eligible for Medicare, Medicaid, or another group health plan, and you have to use up all your COBRA eligibility first.

> ### Bet You Didn't Know
>
> If you've been to the doctor, dentist, or even chiropractor any time in the past couple of years, you received a form to sign regarding the protection of your privacy. Blame (or thank) HIPAA for this form; among it's many requirements, HIPAA also tightened regulations around patient privacy in the medical fields.

◆ State continuation. Most states require companies with fewer than 20 employers to continue health insurance coverage for certain employees and their families under certain conditions. Check with the office of the state insurance commissioner to learn about your state's regulations.

◆ Conversion. Many states let you convert your existing group health coverage into an individual policy with the same insurer. Again it will likely be costly, but at least you'll have coverage.

If you immediately begin a new job with no loss of health benefits, then your new employers' health plan must immediately begin covering you, including any *pre-existing conditions* such as diabetes. This is a federal requirement.

MedLingo

A **high-risk individual** is one who has a pre-existing medical condition, such as diabetes or heart disease, which results in higher medical costs than someone without the condition. They generally have to pay higher premiums than someone with no pre-existing conditions, and might have trouble finding individual coverage. A **pre-existing condition** is a condition for which you have received medical treatment in the past 12 months.

But if there is a gap in your health insurance coverage, for instance, if you didn't take advantage of COBRA and let your health insurance lapse, your new health insurer can exclude coverage of your diabetes for up to 12 months. During this time, you have to pay for your own care. It will also be more difficult to find an individual health policy, if necessary, because you have now become what insurers refer to as a *high-risk* individual.

Bet You Didn't Know

As of May 2004, 46 states have implemented some kind of law requiring health insurance coverage to include treatment for diabetes, according to the National Conference of State Legislatures. That doesn't mean you will be covered; it just means that if you are covered, the health insurer has to cover the cost of your diabetes treatment. The states not included are Alabama, Idaho, North Dakota, and Ohio. To see what's going on in your state, go to the Conference's website at www.ncsl.org/programs/health/diabetes.htm.

I Can't Find (or Can't Afford) Health Insurance

Are you one of the 41.2 million Americans without health insurance? Well, at least there's some slim comfort in numbers. Unfortunately, that's about all there is. Without health insurance, your doctor bills, testing supplies, and medications will eat up a major chunk of your income. That's probably why studies find that many people with chronic conditions such as diabetes who can't afford to pay for their medications wind up cutting back on the amount they take and don't seek medical attention when they should, but wait until things really get bad.

This, of course, is a foolish, dangerous thing to do. It could send you to the hospital with serious complications—and in the long run, it can wind up costing you (and the economy) more.

If you don't have health insurance, or your medications are not covered by your health insurance, you do have several options:

♦ Find a pharmaceutical company low-income program. Most pharmaceutical companies have programs in which they provide medications for free or at a reduced price. See the resources list in the back of this book for specific programs.

♦ Join a high-risk pool. Many states have created programs that offer insurance coverage to people who have been turned down for insurance because of their health. Call your state health insurance commissioner's office, or visit the Georgetown University Health Policy Institute at www.healthinsuranceinfo.net for more information. Unfortunately, the cost for this insurance can be high, but you still might be able to save money over paying everything out of pocket.

♦ Ask your doctor/pharmacist/hospital for a lower fee in exchange for paying in cash. Many will do this because it means that they don't have use their resources to try and collect payments from the insurance company.

♦ See if you qualify for Medicaid, the joint state/federal health insurance program for low-income individuals.

♦ See if you qualify for Medicare. If you're officially disabled, you might be entitled to Medicare coverage, even if you're not 65 or older.

♦ Consider catastrophic health insurance. This is a policy that covers you only if something major happens such as a cancer diagnosis, an automobile accident, or a severe complication of diabetes. With this kind of insurance, the premiums are fairly low, but there is a high deductible, which means you have to pay a lot before the insurance kicks in. After you meet the deductible, however, you're covered. This type of insurance at least protects you from budget-busting healthcare costs that could lead to bankruptcy.

♦ Check with your spouse or domestic partner. Some states allow unmarried individuals living together to cover one another on their health insurance.

> **Bet You Didn't Know**
>
> Recent studies find that medical costs are the leading cause of personal bankruptcy.

◆ Join an association or your local Chamber of Commerce if you have your own business. This is often a good way to find affordable health insurance if you don't qualify for group plan rates.

Medicare: A Good Idea Gone Bad

When President Lyndon Johnson signed the Medicare bill in 1965 to provide health-care coverage for all Americans 65 and older, the medical landscape was a relatively simple one. We knew relatively little about most diseases, had relatively few effective drugs, and the majority of serious care was provided in hospitals.

The few prescription drugs that did exist were fairly affordable, and a visit to your family doctor (generally, the only doctor most Americans saw) cost just a few dollars. And so the Medicare program—groundbreaking legislation in its day—was designed to provide maximum coverage for inpatient hospital care and some coverage for out-patient care, but *no* prescription drug coverage.

Today, Medicare covers 41 million people, 35 million who are over age 65, and another 6 million who qualify on the basis of permanent disabilities. Hundreds of drugs are available for a multitude of conditions, and the average Medicare beneficiary is taking six or more prescription medications at any one time.

Recognizing all that (and helped along by some savvy politicking), the federal government plans to begin providing some prescription drug coverage for Medicare beneficiaries January 1, 2006. That's when the Medicare Modernization Act takes effect.

Before you break out the champagne and toss the confetti, however, note the operative word: *some*. Unless you meet stringent income requirements, you'll have to pay a monthly premium, meet an annual deductible, and pay a portion of your drug cost yourself even with the coverage.

It's far from ideal.

One option is to pay for so-called *Medigap* insurance, supplemental insurance that pays for those things Medicare doesn't. Of course, this will cost you, but it might be worth it to ensure that you can pay for all your medications.

> **MedLingo**
>
> **Medigap insurance** is an insurance policy that covers those things Medicare doesn't pay for such as certain procedures, co-insurance, and other out-of-pocket costs.

Medicaid: Pinched from All Ends

Every state and U.S. territory offers its low-income citizens (primarily pregnant women, children, teenagers, the disabled, the elderly, and the infirm) medical coverage under the Medicaid program. Jointly funded by the federal and state government, this program generally provides comprehensive coverage for most health-related care, ranging from primary care to hospitalization. It also covers long-term care such as nursing homes.

But with rising medical costs and dropping revenues, many states are finding that their Medicaid programs are simply too large a part of their budget. They're raising eligibility requirements to cut the number of people who qualify for Medicaid , and are slashing benefits right and left for the people who are still eligible.

> ### Bet You Didn't Know
>
> As if finding good health insurance when you have diabetes wasn't hard enough, you may also have problems finding a good life insurance policy. The American Diabetes Association (ADA) notes that after you're diagnosed with diabetes, life insurance policies sold within the United States can become "unaffordable or unavailable." Don't get too discouraged. The ADA also notes that some life insurance companies actually specialize in selling policies to people with chronic health conditions like diabetes. It will cost you—but at least you'll have peace of mind that if something happens to you, your loved ones will be protected.

MedLingo

Nonprofit organizations such as the American Diabetes Association and government agencies such as the Agency for Health Care Quality publish **clinical guidelines** that tell doctors the best way to prevent and treat certain conditions based on published research.

It's Up to You: Your Role in Disease Management

Disease management is one of the hottest new terms in the treatment of chronic diseases like diabetes. Technically, it's a system of coordinated care and communication for people whose diseases require a lot of self-care. In other words, it's working as a team with your doctor, diabetes educator, nutritionist, and so on, and making sure you take responsibility for your condition.

Of course, there's a lot more to it, including setting and measuring goals (such as your HbA1c), evaluating how well you and the members of your team are doing in meeting their goals (for instance, one goal for your doctor might be to check your feet during every visit), and improving your access to preventive services and prescription drugs. The medical professionals involved in the program generally develop your treatment based on accepted *clinical guidelines*, a kind of recipe of how to manage diabetes based on well-designed studies.

It's definitely worth it to find a clinic, hospital, or managed care organization that has begun a disease management program for diabetes. Some studies find that such programs can improve blood sugar levels, complications, weight loss, and overall outcomes while potentially reducing costs. Ask your doctor about a diabetes disease management program in your area.

The Least You Need to Know

- You need to work with your doctor to put together a diabetes team to help you manage your disease.

- Your diabetes team should include a physician, diabetes educator, dietitian, and social worker and/or therapist. However, recognize that your health insurance might not cover some of the costs of seeing these professionals.

- It is critical to obtain and keep good health insurance when you have diabetes.

- You do have options if you can't find or afford health insurance.

- A disease management approach is one of the best ways to treat diabetes.

Chapter 5

Exercise Is Everything

In This Chapter

- ◆ The importance of exercise in weight reduction and glucose control
- ◆ Staying safe while exercising
- ◆ Incorporating exercise into your daily life
- ◆ Types of exercise
- ◆ Exercising with diabetic complications

You already know that you're much more likely to have diabetes if you're overweight. The question is why.

It all has to do with the effect that weight has on your cells. Being over-weight or obese increases whatever insulin resistance you've inherited. Plus, the more overweight you are, the more fat cells you have—fat cells stuffed with fatty acids created from excess glucose. In some unknown way, these fatty acids keep insulin from working normally in muscle, fat, and liver. The worst place for this fat? Around your middle, especially your abdomen. The greater the ratio of abdominal fat compared to hip fat, the more insulin resistant you are and the harder time you will have controlling your diabetes.

It's no secret that it takes a combination of diet and exercise to lose weight. In the next chapter, we talk about food and diet. In this chapter, we get up, get moving, and focus on exercise.

Exercise: Everything for Everyone

Even if you're not overweight, exercise can still help you control your blood sugar levels. In fact, using exercise the right way at the right times can even reduce your need for oral medications or insulin! Yet less than a third of people with type 2 diabetes get the recommended amount of daily exercise (about 30 minutes a day, about five days a week). In fact, about a third get *no* regular physical activity at all!

Don't let yourself fall into that category.

Exercise has numerous benefits beyond helping you manage your blood sugar levels. It can prevent depression (or at least help you feel better faster if you suffer from depression), keep your bones strong and help prevent *osteoporosis*, reduce your risk of heart disease (the leading cause of death in people with diabetes), and possibly reduce your risk of some cancers, as well as give you a much needed energy boost.

MedLingo

Osteoporosis is a condition in which your bones become weak and eventually break down, resulting in fractures.

Plus, it can lower your cholesterol levels, help you lose weight, and enable you to reach and maintain a healthier blood pressure. Too bad it can't pay the mortgage and teach your teenager to drive!

What Happens When You Exercise

A lot happens when you exercise. Exercise works in a complex feedback loop that tries to maintain a normal blood sugar range in your body. In people without diabetes, blood glucose concentrations remain normal while you're active because several things happen at once.

- ◆ At the beginning of exercise, the muscle tissues break down glycogen, the stored from of glucose, to use as energy.

- ◆ But the glycogen is rapidly used up, so the muscle tissue starts using glucose from the bloodstream.

- The extra glucose is in your blood because when you start exercising, certain hormones are released, the most important of which are glucagon from the alpha cells of the pancreas (remember that one from Chapter 3?) and *adrenaline* from the *adrenal gland* and nerve endings. These hormones cause the liver to break down its glycogen into glucose and release it into the blood stream.

- On the muscle end, exercise helps your muscles use glucose more efficiently. This helps the glucose concentration in the blood stay normal because the muscles take up the extra amount released by the liver.

- If the exercise is intense enough or lasts long enough, your fat cells start to produce the energy your muscles need by breaking down triglycerides (remember them from Chapter 3?).

MedLingo

Adrenaline is a hormone secreted in times of stress that causes quickening of the heart beat, strengthens the force of the heart's contraction, enables the lungs to take in more oxygen, and has numerous other effects. It is released by the **adrenal glands**, which sit just above the kidneys.

- Here's where it gets good. As your fat cells give up triglycerides, they shrink. Yup, you heard us right. You're losing the fat from your fat cells. Losing fat! In fact, moderate exercise can increase the amount of fat you burn up by tenfold. Yeah!

Now, let's go back to how exercise increases the amount of glucose getting into the muscles. It does this in several ways that we know about, and, probably, several other ways that we don't know about yet. One is that the more you exercise, the greater the number of blood vessels you have supplying your muscles with oxygen and nutrients. The more blood vessels you have heading to muscles, the more glucose can leave your blood stream to be used by that muscle tissue, thus lowering blood sugar.

A second way exercise increases the amount of glucose entering muscles involves the contraction of muscles as you exercise. Remember the glucose transporters that stayed inside muscle cells and went to the surface of the cell to bring glucose in when insulin was around? Well, insulin is just one signal that makes this happen.

It turns out that exercise also has this effect in a way that is altogether independent of insulin. Yes, your muscle cells can turn up their noses at insulin if you're exercising! (For just a bit, anyway). It seems that a signal inside muscle cells is turned on by exercise and triggers glucose transporters to move; unfortunately, we're not quite sure just *how* this occurs.

Some kinds of exercise, such as weight lifting, make the muscle tissue stronger and bigger. That's another reason your body gets better at using glucose. It makes perfect sense if you think about it. Your muscles are one of the biggest users of glucose. The more muscle cells you have, the more glucose your muscles need, and the less leftover glucose remains in your blood!

A Different Picture: Exercising When You Have Diabetes

Now, what happens if you have diabetes? If your insulin is not working effectively (think insulin resistance), then the glucose that your liver releases during exercise builds up in your blood stream, because insulin is still important in getting glucose into muscle cells in addition to the ways in which exercise helps get it there. This results in a high blood sugar level.

However, if you exercise enough, the extra glucose starts getting into your muscle tissue anyway, because of the way in which exercise increases the action of glucose transporters described above.

On the other hand, if you take insulin and exercise a lot without eating a snack, your blood sugar can drop like the proverbial stone Why is this?

Muscle tissue takes up more glucose from your blood because of the exercise. If you've injected insulin shortly before you began exercising that insulin causes even more glucose to enter muscle tissue. But in the midst of all this, insulin blocks any extra glucose from coming from the liver, so your blood sugar drops. That's why you have to be careful when you exercise if you take insulin, especially if you haven't eaten.

The moral of the story is this: work closely with your doctor to figure out the best way to avoid too-high, and especially too-low, blood sugars.

CAUTION Warning

Another type of medication besides insulin can also lead to low blood sugars during exercise. These are the sulfonylurea agents that we talk about in Chapter 7. Because they increase the amount of insulin that your beta cells release, you can have extra insulin available when you're exercising even though you don't need it. Result: hypoglycemia.

Before You Start

Always (that means always, always, always!) check with your doctor first before you begin any kind of exercise program. Ideally, you should have a complete physical evaluation, including a *cardiac stress test* if you're over 40, have risk factors for heart disease besides diabetes, and plan on doing more than mild exercise (mild exercise being a walk around the block or some minor yard work).

If you are taking insulin or a sulfonylurea agent, moderate or intense exercise can cause your blood sugars to get too low. Therefore, you should test before you start exercising. If your levels are below 100 mg/dL when you're about to start your workout, sip on some juice or eat a small piece of candy to increase your levels.

Your doctor should also evaluate you carefully for diabetic neuropathy, as that can affect the type of exercise you can do.

MedLingo

During a **cardiac stress test**, a technician measures how well your heart works while you ride a stationary bicycle or walk on a treadmill. Sensors attached to your chest feed information into a machine, which provides a readout of your cardiac activity.

Starting Slowly

No one expects you to run a five-minute mile. And if that's what you expect of yourself the first time you strap on your running shoes, you will fail miserably. But if you set a five-minute mile as a goal to hit, say, six months from now, that's okay.

Now you have to map out how you're going to get there. That's why we've provided this handy exercise chart. It will help you to track what you're doing and what you need to do to meet your goal (or simply ensure that you get some physical activity every day).

Date	Blood sugar before exercising	Blood sugar after exercising	Type of exercise	Heart Rate	Amount of time	Reward

Notice that last column? Reward? Don't shortchange yourself. Every time you complete your exercise/physical activity for the day, you get a reward. Maybe it's a bubble bath. Maybe it's a 30-minute vegfeast in front of a *Friends* rerun. Maybe it's that new doohicky you've been wanting for your car. Whatever.

Every day, set some kind of goal. If you go seven days in a row with some form of physical activity, make your reward larger. Every month, you get an even larger reward (dinner out, a night with your honey in a romantic inn, a new outfit). You deserve it!

How Much Is Enough?

The question of how much exercise is enough exercise is a common one. For many of us, the idea of exercise conjures up images of an intensive workout that leaves us dripping with sweat, one we have to schedule and plan for and mark off at least an hour of our day for.

We say, hooey!

Your goal should be about 30 to 45 minutes of moderate *aerobic* activity three to five days a week. So what is aerobic exercise? It's simply keeping the same large muscle groups moving for at least 10 minutes at a time. When you do that, they require oxygen for energy, hence the name aerobic.

Bet You Didn't Know

What do we mean when we say light, moderate, or intense exercise? Well, if you don't want to try counting your pulse, try the talking test. Light exercise should increase your heart rate somewhat, but you should still be able to have a conversation with someone without any effort; in fact, you should be able to sing. Moderate exercise means that conversation requires a bit more effort and you definitely can't sing. Intense exercise means that even talking is too difficult. Try to avoid exercising this intensely unless you've trained for it.

MedLingo

Cardiorespiratory fitness is a healthy state of heart and lungs resulting from regular aerobic workouts.

Examples include walking, bicycling, jogging, continuous swimming, and many sports. If you continue an aerobic exercise often enough and at a high-enough intensity, your heart and lungs work much better. This is called *cardiorespiratory fitness*. An added bonus is that insulin also works better. In other words, your insulin resistance decreases, which equals an increase in your insulin sensitivity!

Hitting Your Heart Rate Target

How do you know if you're exercising at a high-enough intensity? As you're exercising, your goal is to hit your *target heart rate* and remain at that level for 20 to 30 minutes. This is important for two reasons: to make sure you're not exercising too hard, which could result in an injury or lead to burn out, and to make sure you're not exercising too wimpily, which means you're just wasting your time and not getting the benefits you're after, such as weight maintenance, weight loss, or cardiorespiratory fitness.

Your target heart rate is 50 to 75 percent of your maximum heart rate. The maximum heart rate is the fastest your heart can beat relative to your age. To calculate your target heart rate, use the following formula:

> 220 (beats per minute) minus your age = your maximum heart rate.

Your maximum heart rate multiplied by the intensity level of the exercise you want (50 to 75 percent) equals your target heart rate. Better check with your doctor to decide on the intensity level.

So if you're a 40-year-old man exercising at an exercise level intensity of 70 percent (which is high), take 220 beats per minute and subtract your age (40) for a maximum heart rate of 180. Now multiply this maximum heart rate by your intensity level (180 x 0.70) and you get 126. That's your target heart rate. Ideally, your heart should be beating 126 times a minute for at least 30 minutes at least three times a week (more often is better) to have an effective aerobic exercise program.

If you'd rather dye your hair purple than do math, log onto the Internet and just punch your age and other information into one of the dozens of handy heart-rate calculators. A good one can be found at http://health.discovery.com/tools/calculators/hrc/hrc.html. You can also follow this handy chart from the American College of Sports Medicine:

Relationship Between Age and Target Heart During Exercise

Age (Years)	Average maximum heart rate (100 percent)	Target heart-rate zone (50–75 percent)
20-30	195	98-146 beats per minute
31-40	185	93-138 beats per minute
41-50	175	88-131 beats per minute
51-60	155	83-123 beats per minute
61+	155	78-116 beats per minute

Of course, the more you exercise and the better shape you get in, the higher your target heart rate should be.

> **Sugar Sense** _____
>
> There are two ways to track your heart rate. You can buy one of those fancy heart-rate monitors and simply listen for the beep. Or you can do things the old-fashioned way.
>
> To take your own heart rate, you need to count the beats of your heart. The best place to do this is at the pulse point just under your ear (also ideal for perfume, but that's another tip).
>
> Put your index and middle fingers lightly on the site just where you feel the beating (just below the angle of your jaw). Starting at zero, count each beat for 10 seconds, and then multiply the tally by six. That's your heart rate. Are you within your target zone?

Exercise, Smexercise; We're Talking Movement!

Forget exercise. That implies kickball games, not getting picked for teams in third grade, jumping jacks, and running around a cinder track, … gym memberships, classes, and marathons. Instead, we're talking about movement. Physical activity. Anything that raises your heart rate well above the couch-potato rate.

We're talking a long walk around the block. Weeding one bed in the garden. Swimming about 20 laps in the pool. Skipping half an episode of *CSI Miami* to work against resistance bands. That can be enough, but do more, and you're on your way to weight loss.

And by the way, you don't have to get that workout in a 40-minute chunk. What about a 10-minute walk before you leave for work, another 10 minutes at lunch, and another 10 or, if you're feeling frisky, 20 minutes when you get home from work? Bam! You've just done your daily allotment, helped your cells use insulin better, and improved your long-term outlook.

Here are some other quick-hit ways to get your daily 30 minutes:

♦ Cut the grass with a push mower.

♦ Walk to the store.

♦ Always park your car and walk into a store/restaurant. Never use the drive-thru.

- Wash your own car.

- Take the stairs, not the elevator or esca-
lator.

- Carry your groceries into the house one
bag at a time.

- Park your car at the far end of the parking lot and walk into the store.

- Get a cordless phone and walk around
your house (putting away laundry, picking up clutter, clearing the dinner table)
whenever you have to make or take a
call. Get a phone with a long range; in
nice weather, take it outside and weed
the garden beds.

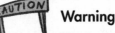

Warning

Always wear a
MedicAlert bracelet, particularly
when you're exercising, and try
not to exercise alone. If you do
go off on a hike, or walk, or
bike ride on your own, make
sure someone knows where you
are. Hypoglycemia can come on
very quickly, leaving you confused and forgetful, possibly
unable to tell anyone your name
or where you live.

And that's only the beginning. You also need to explore unique ways of adding physical
activity to your day, some of which have been studied in terms of their effects on blood
sugar levels. These other possibilities include the following:

- **Swimming:** Other than the bathing-suit issue, swimming is a wonderful activity.
You won't get too hot, the water resistance adds pizzazz to your aerobic routine,
and the quiet of the water and rhythm of the strokes provide a stress-reducing
meditative state.

- **Dancing:** Swing dancing is all the rage now among all ages. Check your newspaper for a swing dancing dance/class near you and sign up. You don't even need a
date; singles come to these events all the time, just looking for someone to twirl.

- **Boxing:** Believe it or not, boxing is one of
the hottest trends in health clubs today.
Again, check the Yellow Pages for a gym
that offers a boxing aerobic class near you.

- **Spinning:** No, we're not talking about
turning around and around until you
throw up. Spinning is a high-intensity aerobic workout performed on special stationary bicycles. You never knew riding a bike
that didn't move could be so much fun!

Bet You Didn't Know

Did you know that you can take
the cost of your gym membership
(and other exercise classes,
equipment, or related expenses)
as a medically related tax deduc-
tion if you're overweight and/or
have diabetes? Ask your doctor
for an exercise "prescription."

Don't try and do the same thing every day. You can get bored, which will give you another reason not to exercise. Instead, alternate workouts. One day, go for a walk. The next day, hit the gym. The following day, go swimming. Another day, walk a different route. You get the picture.

Why Walking Is Best

The best exercise? Walking. It's easy to do, requires no special equipment or training, and can be done anywhere, rain or shine, even while traveling. Plus, it's easy on the joints, provides a good cardiovascular workout, and is, according to scientific studies, the exercise program you're most likely to stick with. The only drawback is that it's not a resistance exercise, so you'll have to add in some form of resistance training for about 20 minutes two or three times a week.

Want to make walking even more fun? Buy a pedometer. These small devices clip onto your waistband and track how many steps you take. People who study such things have come up with the magic number of 10,000 steps a day. It's about 4.5 miles, and it will help you maintain, if not actually lose, some weight (of course, what you eat plays a very important role here, too).

Plus, there's something about the competition—even if you're only competing against yourself to walk more steps than you did yesterday—that can keep you motivated in a way that even rising blood glucose levels might not.

Warning

No matter what form of exercise you choose to follow (unless it's swimming) don't scrimp on your shoes. You learn more about your risk for something called *diabetic neuropathy* and how that can lead to foot problems in Chapter 19, but for now, just understand that any injury to your feet, even something as seemingly simple as a blister, can create a major problem.

So don't buy your shoes at Wal-Mart. Instead, visit a reputable sporting goods shop with trained sales staff. Explain what you're planning to do in terms of physical activity, let the clerk know you have diabetes, and ask for help finding and fitting a quality shoe.

It's also important to replace your shoes regularly. If you're walking a couple of miles a day several days a week, for instance, you should probably replace your shoes every six months or so.

Revving Up Your Walking

If you're worried that you'll get bored while you walk, then try these rev-it-up tips:

♦ Download books on tape onto CDs or your MP3 player and "read" while you walk.

♦ Figure out how many "steps" it would take to get to Paris from your home, and then chip away at the distance day by day. When you finally reach Paris (or even just the town down the road) reward yourself with a fine French meal. (Make sure that you don't do this too often; fine French meals will probably have too many calories and too much fat.)

♦ Download your favorite high-stepping music into your MP3 player and listen to it only when you walk.

♦ When it's errand time, drive into town, and then park your car at the bank and use it as your base to walk to the dry cleaners, sandwich shop, florist, and so on. If you live in the spread-out suburbs, try parking at the far end of the shopping center and using the strip mall as your "town."

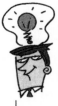

Sugar Sense

How do you feel about dogs? There's nothing like the twin needs of a dog to pee outside and your desire to protect your hardwood floors and carpets to get you up and out the door every morning and evening. If you're allergic, consider joining your neighbor to walk *his* dog. Your neighbor will love you for it and the "task" of walking the dog will give purpose to your exercise beyond improving your blood sugar.

Watching TV While You Work Out

Sure, there's the old, put-the-treadmill-in-front-of-the television-and-sweat thing. But we're talking about something else. How about renting or buying exercise videos, and then spending half an hour or so in front of the tube in your personalized exercise class? The advantage is, you'll never get bored. You can even find videos or DVDs to rent for free from the library. For even more fun, consider inviting a neighbor for a regular session.

Another great at-home exercise idea that requires a television is dance pads. These specially designed floor pads hook up to a video game player. You try to follow the steps on the screen and "beat" your own score. They're guaranteed to get you out of breath.

When You Simply Can't Get Motivated

The hardest part about exercising isn't the exercising. It's the motivation. Look, unless you're a super athlete (in which case, you can skip right over this chapter), a warm bed is always going to look better at 5:30 A.M. than a jog in the gray morning. Vegging on the sofa with the newspaper and a junky rerun is always going to be more appealing than hitting the gym.

The key is to trick yourself into exercising. It's like anything else in life: once you're actually doing it, you'll wonder what all the fuss was about.

To get yourself motivated, try these little tricks:

♦ Keep a pair of walking shoes and athletic socks in the trunk of your car, your office, and by the back door. That way, whenever the urge for fresh air hits, you're ready to go.

♦ Roll out of bed and dress in your workout clothes immediately. Since you're dressed, you might as well work out. If you're not a morning person, change into your workout clothes as soon as you get home from work, even if you think you have no intention of working out.

♦ Work out with a friend. There's nothing like guilt to get you going. If either you or your friend begs off a workout, make a rule that you have to pay $1 into a kitty. At the end of the year, whoever paid the least amount (the one who begged off the least) gets the money.

> **Bet You Didn't Know**
>
> The older you are, the more you need to exercise. A study out of the Mayo Clinic in Rochester, Minnesota, found that the benefits of exercise on reducing insulin resistance in people with diabetes doesn't last as long in people over 65.

Why the Weight You Lift Can Be the Weight You Lose

If the idea of lifting weights puts you in mind of a Mr. (or Ms.) America with bulging pecs and thighs the size of small trees, you need some readjustment in your thinking.

The kind of weightlifting we're talking about merely tones your arms and legs, gives you enough strength to heft that laundry basket up two flights of stairs, and makes it easier to do those seasonal chores that always leave you aching (such as raking leaves, shoveling snow, and washing the car). Oh yeah, did we mention what it will do for your blood sugar levels?

How about improved insulin sensitivity, especially if you're combining it with regular aerobic exercise? In fact, one study found that 4 sets of 12 repetitions of weightlifting added to a 75-minute aerobic class helped a group of postmenopausal women lose the fat around their belly—the so-called toxic fat. That in turn, led to increased insulin sensitivity.

Why? Because resistance exercise builds muscle; the more muscle you have, the more muscle tissue you have to use up glucose.

The Low-Tech Weightlifting Approach

Although it's great if you have a gym where you can work out on resistance machines, a low-tech approach can work just as well. Start with a set of 3-, 5- and 10-pound weights. Put together a 20-minute program that utilizes all the major muscle groups, aiming for slow and steady repetitions at the highest weight you can handle, rather than doing more repetitions at a lower weight. You can call on a personal trainer, a gym instructor, or even find details in a book about resistance training.

Remember, the heavier the weights, the more muscle you're building and fat you're burning. The lighter the weights and more frequent the repetitions, the more endurance you're building.

An added bonus is that because you're building muscle, you're also losing body fat. So even if you don't lose any weight, you might find that once you start a resistance routine, you've lost inches around your body—and dropped a couple of clothing sizes in the process!

Sugar Sense

Keep a pair of 5-pound weights by your desk, by the chair where you watch TV, even in your car. During commercials, spend five minutes doing sit-ups with a weight held across your chest. When you're stuck in traffic, put the car in park and do some arm exercises. Set the alarm on your computer calendar to beep every three hours—your signal to do 15 minutes of crunches.

One caveat is this: Limit major weightlifting sessions (20 minutes or more) to every other day. Your muscles need time to recover between sessions. That soreness you feel is tiny muscle fiber tears resulting from the stretching and unexpected strain.

MedLingo

Anaerobic exercise occurs when the heart rate reaches 50 to 75 percent of the maximum heart rate. **Isometric exercises** involve the application of a force against an immoveable object such as sit-ups, pushups, even pushing against a wall. **Pilates** is a program of stretches and exercises designed to strengthen the core muscles of your back and abdomen.

Resistance Beyond Weights

Lifting weights isn't the only way to get a good *anaerobic* workout. You can get the same benefits by using an exercise ball to practice *isometric exercises*, in which you work against your own body weight.

How about a *Pilates* class, which is designed to strengthen core muscles, such as your abdomen and back? Or try resistance bands, which are oversized rubber bands that you pull and stretch against.

Sit-ups, push-ups, pushing against a wall or desk, lifting gallon jugs of bottled water or milk—all these activities help your muscles move against a resistant object, thus strengthening them.

Exercising with Diabetes-Related Complications

If you think you can use a diabetes-related health condition such as neuropathy, kidney disease, or retinopathy as an excuse not to work out, think again. A recent review of studies found very little evidence that these conditions changed the risks or benefits of exercise. A panel of experts concluded that the risks, if any, were minimal. Specifically, here's what they recommend:

◆ **Retinopathy:** There's no evidence that exercise or physical activity makes your vision or the progression of the mild or moderate form of the eye disease any worse. So, if that's the kind of eye disease you have, get out there and take a jog. If, however, you have a more severe form of retinopathy (your doctor will know), it's probably best that you avoid intense high-impact aerobics (such as tennis or running) or weight resistance activities (such as lifting heavy weights). Instead, consider gentler activities such as bike riding, swimming, or walking.

◆ **Peripheral neuropathy:** If you have this condition, in which there is a reduced sensation in your feet, it makes sense to take it easy on your limbs. Instead of a four-mile hike, consider swimming for an hour, bicycling, or doing upper-body calisthenics.

- **Autonomic neuropathy:** This condition significantly increases your risk of cardiovascular disease and heart attacks, so make sure that you clear any kind of exercise program with your doctor first. He or she might suggest that you sign on for a cardiac rehabilitation program, which is designed for people with heart-related diseases.

- **Kidney disease:** There's no evidence of any harm from physical activity if you have kidney disease. In fact, at least one study suggests that resistance training (weight lifting) might reduce your risk of kidney disease.

The Least You Need to Know

- The more you weigh, the harder time you'll have controlling your diabetes.

- Exercise is an important component of any weight-loss plan, but it can also help you control blood sugar levels even if you're not overweight.

- You should always check with your doctor before beginning any exercise program. If you are taking insulin or a pill called a sulfonylurea agent, you might need to track your blood sugar levels carefully before and after any workout.

- You should aim for a mix of aerobic and resistance exercises each week.

- Walking is one of the best exercises to try.

- Physical activity should become a part of your life, not something you do separately.

Chapter 6

The Food Issue

In This Chapter

- ◆ When to eat
- ◆ How to eat
- ◆ The math behind weight loss
- ◆ Dining out without breaking the calorie bank

As someone with diabetes, you know that you have a high risk of developing various complications, including heart disease, high blood pressure, nerve damage, eye damage, and kidney disease. What and how you eat plays a role in preventing or minimizing these complications.

And just to throw another monkey wrench into your plans for a pizza pig-out this evening, you also have to watch your weight. If you don't maintain a reasonable, realistic body weight, you will need to take more medication, your blood sugar control will be as haphazard as temperatures in March, and you're much more likely to develop the complications that you'll read about later in this book.

Remember the film strips you watched in elementary school? The ones with the dancing bread and apple? The ones that taught you the four food groups? Well, the days of those four food groups are long over. It's time for another lesson in nutrition. Welcome to the world of carbohydrates, protein, and fat. We'll try and keep this simple.

Let's start with the basics.

Coming to Terms with Carbohydrates

Carbohydrates are basically sugars and starches. A teaspoon of sugar? Carb. A potato? Carb. An ear of corn? Carb. With all the low-carb hype, carbohydrates have gotten a bad rap. They're being blamed for everything from the obesity and diabetes epidemic to the extra five pounds you put on last Christmas. We wouldn't be surprised to see them turn up on the Homeland Security list of most-wanted terrorists.

But trying to paint all carbohydrates with the same brush is like saying that anyone who drinks a glass of wine is an alcoholic.

Carbohydrates, whether they come from sugar or starches, are your body's primary source of energy. They're quickly broken down into glucose in your intestinal tract and absorbed into the bloodstream, whether they come from a piece of candy or a high-fiber cereal. They are the nutrient you need to worry about most when it comes to timing meals with taking insulin.

Carbs: Not So Simple

We've gotten used to calling carbohydrates "simple" and "complex." Simple carbohydrates refer to several-sugar molecules attached together, while complex carbohydrates refers to long chains of sugar molecules attached to each other. It turns out, though, that all carbohydrates break down in the intestine to single molecules of glucose for absorption, regardless of how they start out. So even though you might *think* that simple carbohydrates break down faster and raise blood glucose levels more quickly than complex carbohydrates, it just ain't so.

What's more important in terms of a carbohydrate's effect on your blood sugar is how it's cooked, what form it's in (in other words, liquid or solid), and how close it is to its natural state (as opposed to something that more resembles the box it came out of).

That's why the World Health Organization is trying to discourage the use of the terms "simple" and "complex" carbohydrates.

> **CAUTION**
>
> **Warning** _____
>
> Sugar by any other name is still sugar. So beware of the following when you're reading labels; they're all used as nutritive sweeteners and contain about four calories a gram. All can affect your blood sugar levels.
>
> - ◆ Fructose
> - ◆ Levulose
> - ◆ Glucose
> - ◆ Honey
> - ◆ Lactose
>
> - ◆ Maltose
> - ◆ Molasses
> - ◆ Sucrose
> - ◆ Turbinado
> - ◆ Corn syrup

Sugar alcohols (dulcitol, mannitol, sorbitol, and xylitol) contain only two to three calories per gram, but if eaten in high-enough amounts (20 gram portions or 50 grams a day), they can cause diarrhea. However, they are converted to glucose more slowly, require little or no insulin to be metabolized, and don't cause sudden increases in blood sugar.

Nonnutritive sweeteners, like saccharin, aspartame, acesulfame K, and sucralose have no calories and no effect on your blood sugar levels.

An Apple a Day

To better understand the carbohydrate issue, consider the apple, which has 21 grams of carbohydrates. If you eat it whole, your blood sugar rises less and rises more slowly (but stays up longer) than if you take the same amount of carbohydrate in the apple and eat it in the form of apple sauce. But if you drink the same amount of carbohydrate in that apple in the form of apple juice, your blood sugar spikes even higher and faster (but comes down more quickly).

Put those three forms of apple into a meal, however, and whatever else you're eating changes how your body absorbs the carbohydrates, so there's little difference in how the three affect your blood sugar.

A Carb Is a Carb Is a Carb ...

Given all this, any expert in diabetes nutrition will tell you that a carb is a carb is a carb after you eat it. Simple, complex, good, bad—it doesn't matter. If you have diabetes, you have to learn to be aware of the *amount* of carbohydrates you're eating with each meal rather than the *type*, because of the effect they have on blood sugar.

Now, having said all that, we're going to turn around and steer you toward the complex carbohydrates. Why? For several reasons:

◆ Simple carbohydrates, with the exception of plain sugar and fruit, generally come in packages that tend to include fat and be high in calories (such as candy, cookies, pastry, juice).

◆ Complex carbohydrates come packaged with fiber (such as brown rice, whole grain cereal, broccoli). That fiber (more on fiber later) slows your body's absorption of the food, resulting in less-sudden and dramatic effects on your blood sugar.

◆ Complex carbohydrates generally exist close to their natural state; thus they're more nutritionally beneficial because they contain vitamins and minerals along with the aforementioned fiber.

Sugar Sense _____

One of the most common misconceptions about diabetes is that you're not allowed to have sugar. Let's dispel that myth right now. It's not the sugar that's the problem; it's the carbohydrates. If you want to eat chocolate bars for lunch (not something we recommend), you can, as long as you consider the amount of carbohydrates you're getting and the affect it will have on your blood sugar. If you're taking insulin, you can compensate for the extra amount of carbohydrate with additional short- or rapid-acting insulin (more about insulin in Chapter 7). And, of course, you'll need to take into account the extra calories from the chocolate as you total up the number of calories you're supposed to be eating (more on that later, too).

The Glycemic Index: What It All Means

It's likely you've been hearing a lot of talk about something called the *glycemic index*, particularly in relation to where foods fall upon this mythical index. Here's the scoop.

The glycemic index measures how much and how fast certain foods raise your blood sugar levels. Well, actually, it measures how fast the *sugar* in those foods raises levels. This is the kind of thing we discussed earlier for an apple. The apple has the lowest glycemic index, and apple juice has the highest glycemic index.

Now, you know that apple juice is usually sweeter than an apple. So maybe you're figuring, "This glycemic index thing isn't that hard to understand; the sweeter the food, the higher its spot on the index, right?" Not exactly.

The way food affects your blood sugar is a result of several things, not just its sugar content. For instance, as we noted earlier, high-fiber foods result in slower increases in blood sugar because the fiber slows the rate at which you absorb the nutrients. Also as mentioned earlier, how the food is processed and what form it ends up in when you eat it also affects how fast it's absorbed.

So does it make sense, then, that if you have diabetes you should stick to a diet with lots of low-glycemic foods? Well, not exactly. Studies looking at the differences in HbA1c and *fructosamine* levels (tests that provide a glimpse of average blood sugar over time) found no consistent improvements in these tests based on glycemic index diets, and mixed results when it came to levels of blood fat like cholesterol.

The bottom line is, if you follow the kind of diet plan we recommend here, you're going to have pretty good control over your blood sugar levels without worrying about where a particular food falls on some index.

MedLingo

The **fructosamine test** measures how many blood glucose molecules are linked to protein molecules in your blood, providing information on your average blood glucose level for the past three weeks.

What About Low-Carb Diets?

Honestly, the jury is still out on the use of low-carb/high-protein diets for people with diabetes. The studies conducted so far on the use of such diets, which limit the amount of carbohydrates one eats and pumps up the amount of protein, have been small and short. Some studies on low-carb diets showed that they might be helpful; others did not.

Also a direct head-to-head comparison between a low-carb and high-carb/low-fat diet showed no differences when it came to weight loss. Additionally, earlier research found that too much protein in the diet of someone with diabetes could make any existing kidney disease worse.

If you want to reduce the amount of carbohydrates in your diet, that might be fine (as long as your doctor and nutritionist agree). But that doesn't mean you have permission to replace carbs with high-fat foods and skimp on the veggies and fruits. Instead, follow a healthy low-carb diet by following these steps:

- Get rid of all refined carbohydrates, such as white rice, bread, sugary cereals, baked goods, and so on, that don't contain much fiber.

- Nix the sodas and fruit juices (which you shouldn't be drinking anyway).

- Stock up on lean protein sources: eggs, chicken breast, tofu, fish, beans (canned are fine as long as you rinse them off to get rid of the salt).

- Hit the veggie counter. You're looking for leafy green vegetables high in fiber and low in natural sugars such as spinach, kale, and collards. Pick up some broccoli, cauliflower, bagged salads, Brussels sprouts, and so on.

- Stick with berries for your fruits. They're low in sugar and high in fiber.

- Choose whole-grain baked goods, pastas, and cereals. If the word "whole" doesn't appear first in the ingredient list, put it back on the shelf.

Picking Out the Protein

When it comes to protein, you don't have to worry about getting enough. Most Americans already get about 50 percent more than the recommended amount of protein each day. If you have any indication of kidney disease (nephropathy), your doctor might want you to limit your protein intake to about 10 to 15 percent of your daily calories. Otherwise, you can go up to 20 percent.

MedLingo

Saturated fat is a kind of fat found in meat and other animal products. Solid at room temperature, it raises levels of blood cholesterol, resulting in **atherosclerosis,** a chronic health condition in which plaque builds up on the walls of your arteries, increasing your risk of a heart attack or stroke.

What you should focus on, however, is the *type* of protein you eat. Classic animal protein, particularly red meat such as steak, pork, and regular dairy, is high in *saturated fat*, which is a major contributor to the development of *atherosclerosis*, about the last thing you need. So reach instead for other forms of protein such as fish and shellfish, eggs and egg whites, beans, soy products, and white chicken meat.

If you're a big red-meat fan, consider game meats such as buffalo, bison, and venison. They're considerably leaner than cuts from domesticated cattle.

Figuring Out Fats

Fats must love carbohydrates; until the low-carb craze came around, fats were the bad guy in the nutritional world. Enter high-protein diets and it seemed at first that the more fat you ate, the more weight you'd lose.

Thankfully, we're beginning to return to our senses in this country, which means returning to an understanding of the dangers of too much fat.

First—and there's no getting around this—fat is more calorically dense than either protein or carbohydrates. Sounds complicated, but what it really means is that there are nine calories in one gram of fat, compared to four in a gram of carbohydrate or protein. Eat a teaspoon of fat and you get about 38 calories; eat a teaspoon of sugar or a teaspoon of soybeans and you get about 16 calories.

Remember, it all comes down to calories; the more calories you get—regardless of where you get them from—the more weight you'll gain unless you're burning those extra calories.

We're not telling you to avoid fat altogether. Fat serves numerous important nutritional purposes: it helps you feel full, it keeps your skin moist and your hair healthy, and it contributes to the production of important hormones. The problem is, you, like most people in this country, are probably getting too much fat in your diet.

So not only do we want you to limit the amount of fat you get (to about 30 percent of your calories), but we want you to choose the right fat in the right amount.

There are three primary kinds of fat you should be concerned with:

1. Saturated fat

2. Unsaturated fat

3. Trans fats

All fats contain a bit of each; it's the proportion that determines their category.

Staying Away from Saturated

Let's start with saturated fat. This is the kind, as we noted earlier, found primarily in animal products. The only other place you'll find them is in palm and coconut oils, the so-called tropical fats.

One easy way to tell if a fat is saturated or not is if it's solid at room temperature. You only have to see what happens to the grease left in the pan after frying up a couple of burgers to know that the fat in that ground beef was saturated.

Saturated fat contributes to heart disease more than any other fat except trans fat. It does this by raising levels of bad cholesterol, called LDL cholesterol. We talk more about this more in Chapter 16. For now, suffice it to say that you should limit the amount of saturated fat to 10 percent or less of your daily calories. If you eat the kind of lean protein we recommend, that shouldn't be difficult.

Unsaturated Fats: The Good and the Bad

Unsaturated fats are just what they sound like. They're not as saturated with hydrogen molecules (more than you wanted to know, we know) as saturated fat, so they remain liquid at room temperature. Olive oil, corn oil, vegetable oil, walnut oil—they're all unsaturated. That doesn't mean you can gulp them down. They're still fats and full of calories. And within the unsaturated category, there's *monounsaturated* (the good guys) and *polyunsaturated* (the not-so-good guys).

MedLingo

Monounsaturated fats are vegetable oils and fatty acids whose molecular structure includes only one double carbon bond; **polyunsaturated fats** are vegetable oils whose molecular structure has numerous double or triple bonds in a molecule. Monounsaturated fats are generally the healthiest form of fats.

Americans get way more polys (our little nickname) in our diet than we do monos. And it's the monos, research finds, that can help protect you against heart disease. They do this by lowering levels of LDL cholesterol and raising levels of the "good" kind of cholesterol, HDL. Polys, on the other hand, lower LDLs somewhat; but they also drag down the HDLs right along with them.

So when you're reaching for the oil, stick with olive oil, canola, and nut oils like walnut or macadamia. Try to limit the amount of vegetable oils such as corn oil and plain ol' vegetable oil.

Omega-3 Fatty Acids

Okay, as if you weren't confused enough, we now tell you about another type of fat. It technically belongs in the polyunsaturated family, but it's a type of poly that we encourage you to get. It's an essential fatty acid; essential because your body can't manufacture it and thus relies upon the food you eat to get it.

What is this type? Omega-3 fatty acids, found primarily in fatty fish (think mackerel, salmon, and anchovies) and some nuts and seeds such as flaxseed. This type of fat helps protect against *oxidation*, a process that damages cells and leads to disease (more on that in Chapter 10).

It also makes red blood cells more slippery, so they're less likely to clog up arteries and lead to heart disease. Numerous studies find that it has particular benefits for people with diabetes, helping to lower levels of another dangerous blood fat, triglycerides.

MedLingo

Oxidation is a process by which a form of oxygen becomes attached to a molecule, making it chemically unstable and resulting in cellular damage.

Trans Fats

Okay, these are the really bad boys of the fat world. They're the ones who would just as soon take you out in a back alley and shoot you as shake your hand. They're unsaturated fats that have been chemically altered to remain solid at room temperature.

When fats are changed in this way, they increase cholesterol levels and significantly raise your risk of heart disease. In fact, the National Academy of Sciences has concluded that these fats are as bad as, if not worse than, saturated fat in raising heart disease risk. The only safe amount to eat, another government agency found, is none.

The good news? It's gotten much easier to steer clear of these bad guys. As of January 2006, manufacturers are required to list the amount of trans fats on food labels. So read those labels!

Fabulous Fiber

Fiber isn't actually a nutrient because you can't digest it and your body doesn't need it to survive. But you do need it to survive *well*. Fiber is the indigestible plant parts that come in with foods such as whole grains, real fruits, and fresh or frozen veggies (the canned stuff has little, if any).

Why is it so important? Gosh, there are so many reasons. Where to start …

- ◆ Fiber fills you up, not out. That means it makes you think you're full because it fills your stomach, but because you don't digest it, no calories are involved.

◆ Fiber keeps you, how shall we put this, regular. It's a major player in your ability to go to the bathroom when you need to.

◆ Fiber slows the rate at which glucose is absorbed into your blood stream. Think of it as a kind of strainer lined with a coffee filter; everything takes longer to go through. This is particularly important when you have diabetes because it helps you to avoid the peaks of high blood sugar after meals and the troughs that often follow when the immediate dose of glucose ends.

Ideally, you should aim for at least 25 grams of fiber a day (30 is even better).

Exchange Food Programs and Beyond!

So just how do you track what and when you eat? How do you know how many carbs you're getting as well as how much fat? You've got lots of options. We briefly note the primary diabetes "diets," along with the pros and cons of each. We do not, however, tell you which one is best for you. As we've already said (but it bears repeating), only your doctor and nutritionist can determine that. Of course, you have the final say because you're the one who ultimately decides what goes into your mouth (and whether it ends up on your hips or not).

Exchange Diets

In this diet, all foods are assigned to one of six food categories, or *exchanges* (milk, fruit, fat, protein, starch/bread, vegetable). Depending on how many calories you're supposed to get each day, you're told how many exchanges you can have at each meal. For instance, breakfast might be two starch exchanges (each the equivalent of a slice of bread), two fruit exchanges, and one fat exchange. Some foods, such as tea, are "free" exchanges, meaning that you can have all you want.

The pros of this diet are that as long as you can count, you can follow it. If you limit the number of prescribed calories, you're likely to lose weight. Plus, it can help with blood glucose control. It also provides a variety of foods to choose from each day and makes meal planning fairly easy. It just takes a little study to become familiar with what's in each exchange.

Constant Carbohydrate

This program is built around the idea that you should eat a set amount of carbohydrates each day. It differs from the exchange meal plan in that you don't count all types of food; you just count carbs, because carbohydrates have the greatest effect on your blood glucose levels. So you're allotted a certain number of carbohydrates for each meal, with each portion size equaling 15 grams of carbohydrates.

One major pro of this plan is that it's easy to use and track—you only have to worry about one type of food. A con is that if you focus only on carbs, you might wind up shortchanging yourself nutritionally. After all, this plan enables you to get your carbs from any carbohydrate—be it a candy bar or a bowl of brown rice. The number of calories varies depending on the food source of the carbs.

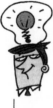

> **Sugar Sense**
>
> Want an easy, high-fiber way to stabilize blood sugar levels? Studies find that just half a cup of beans a day can help stabilize your blood sugar levels. Keep cans of beans in your pantry, and then rinse and sprinkle on salads, mix into tomato sauce, and serve over whole-grain pasta, puree and add to soups, or blend with some lemon juice and garlic for a great appetizer dip (try fresh veggies as the dipper!)

Counting Carbohydrates

This meal plan is designed for those taking insulin. It enables you to balance your insulin dose against the amount of carbohydrates you eat. You still count carbohydrates in 15-gram portions, as with the Constant Carbohydrate plan, but you and your doctor work out how many units of short-acting insulin you need for each carbohydrate exchange you eat.

So for instance, if you eat a cup of frozen yogurt that has 45 grams of carbohydrates, that's three carb exchanges. If you need one unit of insulin for each carb exchange, you would take three insulin units before eating.

The pros of this diet are that it allows more flexibility in what you eat; but the cons are that it can be more difficult to follow because it requires close attention to match what you're eating with how much short-acting insulin you should inject before each meal.

So What *Should* I Eat?

In the old days, diabetes experts used to issue blanket nutritional statements for people with diabetes. There was even an official American Diabetes Association diet. This set limits on how many calories you got, how many servings you ate of different foods, and so on. The problem was, it was the same for everyone!

> **Sugar Sense**
>
> For a fragrant way to maintain blood sugar levels, consider sprinkling cinnamon over your coffee, yogurt, cereal, and tea. Researchers from Pakistan, the birthplace of cinnamon, found that people with type 2 diabetes who took between 1 and 6 grams per day of cinnamon for 40 days had blood glucose levels 18 to 29 percent lower than those who didn't take any cinnamon (in other words, the more cinnamon, the lower their blood sugar levels). Other studies from the US Agricultural Research Service (ARS) found cinnamon seems to make fat cells more responsive to insulin, possibly via a substance within the spice that prevents the oxidative stress.

Today, experts recognize that diabetes is as individual as the person who has it. Therefore, diet plans need to be individualized as well. Still, the major diabetes organizations such as the American Diabetes Association (ADA) and the American Association of Clinical Endocrinologists do issue guidelines every year or so to provide some direction to physicians and patients.

The experts who come up with these guidelines don't just make them up off the top of their heads; they go through all the recent studies and come up with their recommendations based on the best science.

The one thing all that agree on is this: weight loss and maintenance of weight loss in people who are overweight or obese is critical in decreasing the insulin resistance that is the hallmark of type 2 diabetes. Even if you're not actively losing a lot of weight, experts note, simply taking in fewer calories than you're expending will lead to some weight loss and help improve blood glucose levels.

The latest guidelines were issued in 2004. Here's what they recommend:

◆ Stick to foods containing carbohydrates from whole grains, fruits, vegetables, and low-fat dairy.

◆ Remain aware of how many carbohydrates you're getting more than the type you're getting.

◆ Get less than 10 percent of your overall calories from saturated fat (even less if you have a high level of bad cholesterol).

◆ Limit the amount of cholesterol you get from your diet to less than 300 mg/day (about the amount in a small hamburger patty).

◆ If you're taking insulin, you should eat a consistent amount of carbohydrates from day to day at each meal (unless you count carbohydrates, as we discussed previously).

◆ Make sure to get enough fiber in your diet (national guidelines call for 25 grams a day).

◆ You can eat foods that contain sugar (and, for that matter, table sugar itself) as part of a healthy diet.

◆ Minimize the amount of trans fats in your diet.

◆ Keep polyunsaturated fats to about 10 percent of calories.

◆ Limit alcohol consumption to one drink for women and two a day for men. Make sure that you don't drink a lot of alcohol without eating because it can cause low blood sugar (more on alcohol later).

Sugar Sense _____

Don't let the color of bread fool you into thinking that it's whole grain. Some manufacturers add molasses to color white bread, and then try to pass it off as whole grain. Always check ingredient lists before buying.

Still pretty vague, isn't it? Well, we're just giving you the picture from 50,000 feet up. That's why it's so important to include a nutritionist on your treatment team. He or she can devise an individualized nutrition program designed to take into account your weight, age, physical activity levels, and any other medical problems you may have such as high blood pressure or high cholesterol levels.

Timing Is Everything (in Some People)

Now let's talk a bit about *when* to eat. If you're not taking insulin or oral medications in the *sulfonylurea* class, you can skip this part. Otherwise, listen up, because your entire life is now one big balancing act between insulin, food, and blood sugar.

MedLingo

Sulfonylureas are a class of oral diabetes drugs that work by stimulating the pancreas to produce more insulin.

You can't just wake up in the morning and stumble through your day eating whatever you want whenever your stomach starts growling or you smell a Cinnabon stand. You have to have a plan—a meal plan. Think of it as your very own yellow brick road. Follow it throughout the day, and at the end of the day you'll reach the safety of controlled blood sugar levels, that is, levels that neither shoot up too high nor drop too low.

The secret to using insulin safely and effectively is to eat an appropriate diet in a fairly consistent way and to take the appropriate types and amounts of insulin to control the blood sugar. In other words, fit the insulin (which we talk more about in Chapter 8) around the right diet, rather than fit the diet around the insulin.

If you eat erratically, however, it will be very difficult for the insulin to control your blood sugars well. The same is generally true for the sulfonylurea agents, but there you don't have to be as consistent; there's more flexibility in the timing and consistency of your diet.

Playing the Weight-Loss Card

You'd think that if you knew you had diabetes, and you knew that eating a healthy diet and maintaining a healthy weight were about the most important things you could do to stay healthy, that you'd eat right and watch the weight, right?

Why do the majority of Americans with type 2 diabetes still eat a diet high in saturated fat, and get far fewer than the recommended five servings a day of fruit and veggies? Why, then, are 80 percent of Americans with type 2 diabetes still overweight, even after their diagnosis?

Although there are several reasons so many people with diabetes are overweight, the most important one is probably this: it's not easy to change the way you eat.

After all, you've eaten a certain way most of your life, choosing this way of eating because you liked it. Now someone comes along and says you have to change. Is it any wonder that most people feel like saying, "No way, José. I feel okay, why should I change?"

Follow the Three Commandments

The reality is that there is no one "best diet," not even for people with diabetes. Instead, any meal plan you and your healthcare team come up with needs to be built around these three commandments:

1. The fewer calories you eat and the more calories you burn (regardless of where those calories come from), the more weight you'll lose.

2. The more carbohydrates you eat, the higher your blood sugar spikes after a meal.

3. The more saturated fat you get in your diet, the higher your levels of "bad" cholesterol will be, increasing your risk of heart disease.

> **Sugar Sense**
>
> Next time you're planning pasta for dinner, switch to soba. Soba noodles are made with buckwheat, which is high in fiber and known to reduce blood sugar levels. Not into noodles? Try some buckwheat pancakes for breakfast tomorrow.

Losing Weight: It Doesn't Take Much

Now onto one of the most important parts of this chapter—indeed, of this book: How to lose weight. Start with these two steps:

♦ Stop thinking about weight loss in terms of the number of pounds you need to lose.

♦ Stop focusing on the scale.

Start with where you are. Losing just 5 to 10 percent of your weight could make a tremendous difference in your blood sugar control and the risk of complications from diabetes. In fact, it might even be enough to enable you to control your diabetes with exercise and diet alone—no pills or needles for a while. If you weigh 250 pounds, for instance, losing just 5 percent of your body weight—only 12.5 pounds—can make a big difference.

No, it probably won't give you back your 25-year-old waist, but it will provide a realistic goal that will still show substantial results. And it won't take long: a pound or two a week is considered a healthy weight-loss goal. At that rate, it will only take about six to eight weeks to shed the weight.

When you look at it that way, it doesn't seem too onerous, does it?

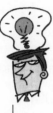

> **Sugar Sense** _____
>
> Get one of your daily fruit servings via a grapefruit. When California researchers asked 50 obese patients to eat half a grapefruit with each meal for 12 weeks and compared them to a group that didn't eat the citrus fruit, they found that those getting the grapefruit lost an average of 3.6 pounds more than the placebo group, and also had lower levels of insulin and glucose after each meal.

The Weight-Loss Equation

There's really only one way to lose weight and keep it off. Ready?

Eat less and move more.

There. Simple, isn't it? There's no getting around it. Your body needs the calories, or energy, in food to survive. For most people, if you're taking in about the same amount of calories as you're burning every day, then you don't know the meaning of the word "overweight." Unfortunately, few of us follow this equation. Instead, we're more likely to follow the equation of eat what we want, sit on the couch, and watch the numbers on the scale.

So how many calories a day do you need? Your doctor or dietitian should be able to tell you (but trust your dietitian/nutritionist more; most doctors are not well trained in nutrition). It depends on your age, weight, and activity level.

The nonprofit Calorie Control Council (yes, they count calories) estimates that someone who is moderately active, meaning that you get about 30 to 60 minutes of exercise at least three times a week, needs about 15 calories per pound of weight to *maintain* that weight. So if you're a 150-pound woman who is moderately active, that's about 2,250 calories a day. But if you are five feet tall and weigh that much, you are way overweight. On the other hand, if you are five feet, ten inches tall, you're right on target. How is all of that figured out?

Getting Your Pound of Fat

One more number to throw at you (and a pretty sobering one). One pound of fat contains 3,500 calories. Every time you accumulate 3,500 extra calories that you don't burn off, you gain a pound of fat. Alternatively, it takes a caloric deficit of 3,500 calories (that is, 3,500 more calories used up than taken in) to lose a pound of fat.

In general, eating 10 or fewer calories per pound of DBW (dietary body weight) leads to a caloric deficit of about 500 calories a day. Therefore, in one week (if you stick to that formula), you should have one pound less of fat on your frame.

How do these numbers translate into the real world? Consider, for instance, that few Americans are active; in fact, the average American woman burns just 1,600 to 1,700 calories a day, yet consumes about 1,900 calories a day. Over a year, that adds up to an extra 20 pounds a year.

On the other hand, if you cut just 100 extra calories a day (about the amount in a four Hershey kisses, four pieces of pepperoni, or 10 fast-food fries), you'll lose a pound a month, or about 10 pounds a year, without even trying. Cut 200 calories a day (about the amount in a can of soda or two tablespoons of butter) and you'll double your weight loss.

Sugar Sense

It's easy to cut calories without even noticing. For instance ...

- ◆ Steam veggies and chicken in broth instead of sautéing in fat. Calories saved are about 200.
- ◆ Switch from regular to diet soda. Calories saved are about 180 per can.
- ◆ Use sugar-free jam on your toast in the morning instead of butter or margarine. Calories saved are about 100.
- ◆ Use skim milk instead of regular. Calories saved are about 110 per cup.
- ◆ Switch to low-cal salad dressings. Calories saved are about 100 in 2 tablespoons.
- ◆ Substitute two egg whites for every whole egg in recipes. Calories saved are about 100 per egg.
- ◆ Order your burger plain. Calorie savings are about 100 per ounce of cheese.
- ◆ Skin the chicken before eating. Calories saved are about 100.
- ◆ Choose low-fat mayonnaise. Calories saved are about 100 per 2 tablespoons.
- ◆ Choose a veggie burger instead of beef. Calories saved are about 200.

But if you have type 2 diabetes, you don't want to wait a year to lose those 10 pounds. That's why following the 10-calories-per-pound-of-DBW rule is important; you'll lose those 10 pounds in 10 weeks. Actually, you'll lose more, but it won't be fat.

Whenever you cut back on carbohydrates, your body first ditches any extra water. On the other hand, if you're on a weight-loss diet and you binge on carbohydrates, you'll gain more weight than just those 3,500 extra calories a pound would put on, because your body is retaining water.

The good news is that it's not fat. So when you return to your weight-loss diet, you'll lose the extra water weight quickly.

How Much Is Enough?

Studies find that successful, long-term weight loss in people with diabetes works best if you cut your calories by between 250 and 500 a day (10 calories per pound of DBW gives about a 500-calorie deficit a day), take in less fat (particularly saturated fat), and increase your physical activity (time to reread Chapter 5). We've already given you some easy ways to cut the calories. What other methods have been shown to work when it comes to weight loss?

- Eat smaller, more frequent meals instead of getting all your calories in three big meals. This helps you to maintain steadier blood sugar/insulin levels throughout the day with fewer peaks and valleys. Note the word "smaller," however. If you're used to having a turkey sandwich and salad for lunch at noon, for instance, have half the turkey sandwich and half the salad around 11 A.M., and then finish off the rest around 2 P.M.

- Keep a journal. No, not the kind with the lock and key; the kind in which you record everything that passes between your lips during the day. Studies find that people who maintain nutritional diaries are more likely to lose weight and keep it off, eating about 15 percent fewer calories a day than those who don't.

- Eat slowly. You probably remember your mother telling you this; well, she was right. It takes about 20 minutes for the signal to pass from your stomach to your brain, telling your brain that you're full. If you gulp your meal in 10 minutes, you might still *feel* hungry, when in reality you're already full and don't need any more calories. Try putting your fork down between each bite or getting up and walking around the table after every five bites.

- Eat your salad first. High in volume but low in calories, a big salad will help you feel full on fewer calories. Another good option is to have a bowl of broth-based (not cream-based) soup before dinner.

- Don't skip breakfast. Studies find that people who eat a healthy breakfast every morning, particularly high-fiber, low-fat cereal, are less likely to be overweight and less likely to get diabetes in the first place.

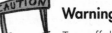

Warning

Turn off the television while you're eating. A study of college students found that participants ate more often and more each time when they watched TV while eating.

Cheers to You, Too!

So we've covered dinner. What about that nice bottle of Bordeaux you've been saving for a special occasion? Can you drink when you have diabetes?

Well, that's really going to be for you and your doctor to decide. But here's what we know about alcohol and diabetes.

There are several effects of alcohol on glucose control in people with diabetes. It depends not only on what you're drinking and how much, but on what you're eating and when you last ate. For instance, because alcohol is processed in the liver, it can interfere with the liver's ability to produce glucose, which could, in turn, lead to hypoglycemia. This is only a problem if you skip meals and drink.

Sugar Sense

Next time you pass a mound of glistening red cherries, stuff a pound in a bag. A study published in the *Journal of Agricultural and Food Chemistry* found that anthocyanins, a class of plant pigments responsible for the color of many fruits, including cherries, might help lower blood sugar in people with diabetes. Don't eat the whole pound at a time, however, and stay away from those bright red maraschino cherries. They've had all the healthful benefits processed out of them and a bunch of sugar added in.

But it's particularly a concern if you're taking insulin or a sulfonylurea. Alcohol can also make triglyceride levels worse. Plus, alcohol still has calories. Remember that fat has nine calories a gram, about twice as much as carbohydrate and protein. Well, alcohol, with 7 calories per gram, has almost as many calories as fat. This comes to about 148 in a can of beer, 106 in a glass of wine, and about 100 in a typical vodka martini. Those extra calories do one thing: they add weight, which makes your diabetes harder to control.

Dining Out with Diabetes

All this information on what to eat and when to eat and how to eat is all well and good when it comes to dining at home; but what about when you're eating out?

Dining out has become a common pastime in this country, one that plays a large role (pun intended) in our expanding waistlines. Studies find that we eat an average of three meals a week prepared outside of the home, and 30 percent of Americans say that meals eaten at a restaurant or fast food establishment are essential to the way they live. Who has time to cook?

But even though eating out has become routine in our lives, we still view it as a special treat and give ourselves permission to order things we'd never eat at home, such as french fries, milkshakes, supersize sodas, and molten chocolate desserts.

No wonder study after study shows that we tend to eat more when we eat out. Today, a small order of french fries typically contains about 200 calories and 10 grams of fat, and a large hamburger has nearly 600 calories and 35 grams of fat. Are you surprised that 60 percent of Americans say they feel it's harder to lose weight when eating out, and 35 percent believe that "all fast food is junk?"

There is hope, however. The growing obesity epidemic has resulted in somewhat of a backlash against the restaurant industry, which in turn is beginning to offer healthier choices on its menus. The key is making the right choice.

Finding Hidden Gems in Fast Food

Today, every fast-food outlet worth its drive-through offers up a delectable selection of salads that are actually large enough to fill you up. Be careful, though. If you add the fried chicken, the croutons, cheese, and regular dressings to some of these salads, you might as well have had a Big Mac and supersized the fries.

Instead, follow these easy tips for maintaining your blood sugar levels while eating out the fast-food way:

♦ Get the chicken broiled, not fried, whether on a sandwich or a salad.

♦ Skip all spreads and dressings unless they're low- or no-fat.

♦ Remember that even ketchup is loaded with sugar, so watch out if you're doing a lot of dunking.

♦ Get out of your car and order and eat in the restaurant. Not only will you burn a few more calories, but you're also more likely to order non-car-friendly foods such as baked potatoes with broccoli, salads, veggie wraps, and chili.

♦ Never, ever "supersize" anything.

Hitting the Sit-Down Chains

Sometimes it seems that chain restaurants such as Applebees, TGI Friday's, Olive Garden, and Bennigans are as ubiquitous as the golden arches. Just consider the numbers. Today, there are nearly 200,000 "table-side" restaurants in the United States, a figure that continues to grow. Like fast-food outlets, these dining establishments can be ticking time bombs when it comes to good nutritional health.

But you're in luck. Nearly all the chains have added healthier options to their menus for those seeking lower amounts of fat and calories in their selections, such as Applebee's Weight Watchers options, Chili's "It's Your Choice" program, which encourages diners to customize their orders, or Red Lobster's "Lighthouse Menu."

Even if your favorite eatery doesn't offer such options, the following tips will help you get out with your blood sugar levels steady, your waistband comfortably loose, and enough leftover food for lunch the next day.

♦ Ask for a doggie bag with your order. Restaurant portions are huge; by putting half into a box right away, you won't be tempted to "clean your plate."

♦ Stay away from anything described as "crunchy, fried, or creamy." Those are all synonyms for "full of fat."

♦ Skip dessert.

♦ Consider making an appetizer your main course. Most of them are more than large enough. But forget about the fried mozzarella and stuffed potato skins.

- Ask for a side salad or some steamed veggies in place of fries, rice, or baked potato.

- Watch out for the salad bar! Anything sitting in any kind of liquid should be off limits. Only choose items that haven't changed from their original state (broccoli, not broccoli salad, for instance).

The Least You Need to Know

- You need to maintain a healthy weight to live healthily with diabetes.

- There is no single "meal plan" for people with diabetes.

- For blood sugar, count carbohydrates—regardless of the type.

- For weight, count calories—regardless of the fancy gimmicks or popular diets.

- You can eat out without busting the calorie bank.

Chapter 7

Time to Pop a Pill

In This Chapter

◆ Medication for diabetes

◆ The importance of your pharmacist

◆ Using medication safely

◆ The five classes of oral diabetes medications

If you had type 1 diabetes, you wouldn't even be reading this chapter. That's because there's only one type of medication prescribed for type 1 diabetes—insulin. Without it, you would die because your body isn't making any insulin on its own. It's a simple as that. But when you have type 2 diabetes, you have more options, including oral medication.

In this chapter, we cover what you need to know about diabetes medications, the drugs themselves, how and when to take them, their pros and cons, and how you can better cope with taking medication. We even give you some tips on developing a better relationship with your pharmacist (hint: flowers never hurt).

Remembering the Basics of Type 2 Diabetes

Before we get too far into the different options, however, let's take a moment for a brief review of what goes wrong when you have type 2 diabetes. It all plays into the issue of medications.

Instead of making you go back and reread Chapter 3, we've got the Cliff Notes version right here:

◆ Most people with type 2 diabetes have insulin resistance, which means that your muscle and liver cells don't respond normally to the insulin your pancreas puts out.

◆ Your pancreas isn't putting out enough insulin to overcome this insulin resistance. As a matter of fact, when your disease is first diagnosed, your pancreas is producing only about half the amount of insulin it should.

◆ As your disease progresses, your sugar levels before and after meals get worse. That's because your liver starts providing too much glucose, ignoring signals from the insulin that tell it to slow its glucose production.

Much of how you'll respond to treatment depends on how long you've had diabetes. That's because your pancreas produces less and less insulin over time. Because high blood sugars don't cause symptoms until they get very high, most people have had type 2 diabetes for years before they are diagnosed. So how you respond to medication depends on how much insulin you have left. If there's not much, you'll need a lot of pills, or even insulin for treatment. On the other hand, if your doctor caught your disease early and you still have a fair amount of insulin left, you might not need any medications, at least for a while, and instead, you can control your disease with diet and exercise.

When diet and exercise alone stop working, however, there's the question of which type of medication you need: an oral medication, called an *oral hypoglycemic agent*, or injectable insulin. If your pancreas is still making some insulin, most doctors will probably start you on an oral drug first. And that's a good thing, because no one likes needles.

> **Bet You Didn't Know**
>
> About 20 percent of people with type 2 diabetes can control their condition with diet and exercise only, sometimes for years.

> **MedLingo**
>
> A **class** of drugs is composed of several individual medications that all work in the same way but may be broken down in the body differently and have different side effects.

Which brings us to the crux of this chapter: which oral drug is best for you? With five different *classes* of oral medication to choose from, about 15 medications overall, and various combinations of drugs that can be used, figuring out which works best for you can be challenging.

Medication? Me? Fuggedaboudit!

No, you can't. No matter how you feel about taking medication—whether a pill or an injection—you should still be thankful that you have such excellent medications available today for the treatment of diabetes. Just remember, as recently as 70 years ago, a diagnosis of diabetes was a death sentence. After your pancreas stopped making insulin, or making enough insulin, you were heading in only one direction—down and out.

Today, however, there are numerous options. We focus on oral medications in this chapter; in the next chapter, we talk about insulin.

You'll know you need medication if you are no longer able to control your blood sugar levels with diet and exercise alone. Of course, this is a decision that you can only make together with your doctor. Also, just because you start on an oral medication doesn't mean that you have to stay on it. Sometimes, losing weight, changing your diet, and/or increasing your physical activity can affect your blood sugar levels to the extent that you no longer need to take medication.

Bet You Didn't Know
Even after you're on insulin, you might be able to eventually return to oral medications or use less insulin in combination with oral medications. Of course, this usually depends on your commitment to diet, exercise, and losing weight.

Welcome to the Wonderful World of Drugs

It's not Disneyland, that's for sure. Now that you're on medication, you have to monitor yourself for side effects, coordinate your medicine with your meals and exercise (depending on what you're taking), and jack up the communication level with your doctor.

Don't Forget to Take Your Medicine

Here's the first rule: take your medicine.

Sounds obvious right? Well, consider that studies find that many patients with diabetes take less than the prescribed medication, whether oral medications or insulin. One study of patients with type 2 diabetes found that those studied took only 63 percent of their doses as prescribed. Two other studies found that the less often people with diabetes took their prescribed medications, the more likely they were to end up in the hospital, resulting in higher healthcare costs and more complications.

MedLingo

Prescription **compliance** refers to taking your medications as directed.

Sustained release refers to a medication in which the active ingredient is released very slowly, enabling you to take just one dose a day.

You're more likely to adhere to your medication regimen when you have to take fewer drugs and take them less often. That's why more drug companies are coming out with once-a-day pills for people with diabetes and combining two types of oral diabetes medication into one pill. They're hoping to improve *compliance*. So ask your doctor if there is a way to streamline the medications you take. You might be able to get a *sustained release formulation* or take all your medications (in addition to your diabetes drugs) at the same time, usually before meals.

Sugar Sense

Try these tips to remember to take your medicine (even without the proverbial teaspoon of sugar!):

♦ Keep your medicines together in one place prominently displayed where you can see them, like near your toothbrush or the refrigerator (obviously, keep them out of reach of any children). Some diabetes medications have to be taken before meals, so an obvious place in the kitchen is another good idea.

♦ Set the alarm on your watch, computer, cell phone, or personal digital assistant to beep when it's time to take your medication.

♦ Make a chart or have a pharmacist make a chart of each medication and the times at which you should take it. Hang the chart on the refrigerator door.

♦ Get a pill box with room for a week's worth of medication. If you have to take pills several times a day, get a separate pill box for each time; for example, one for before breakfast, one for before supper and one for at bedtime. Fill the compartments every Sunday night.

Why does it matter if you're not taking your medicine as prescribed? Beyond the immediate difficulty in controlling your blood sugars, blood fats, and blood pressure (which will eventually lead to complications and higher healthcare costs) there are other repercussions. Your doctor might assume that you're undermedicated and pre-scribe a larger dose. Or your doctor might start switching your medication to try to find one that works better. This is annoying, cumbersome, expensive, and potentially dangerous—particularly if you don't take the new medication as prescribed, either.

There's No Magic Bullet

Here's the second rule on pill taking: they are not a magic bullet. They do not excuse you from watching your diet and exercising. They do not mean that your illness is going to go away. And just because you're not taking insulin does not mean that you do not still have a serious illness.

Plus—and this is really important—taking your pills does not mean that you can test your blood sugar less frequently than your doctor asked you to. They also aren't optional; just because you're feeling well or because your blood sugar levels are test-ing normal doesn't mean you can skip a dose of medicine.

> **CAUTION**
>
> **Warning** _____
>
> Are you taking too many medications? It's quite likely. Studies find that older people (and you're more likely to have diabetes if you're over 50) make up about 13 percent of the population, but consume about one third of all prescription medications, with most taking several at a time. It's called *polypharmacy*, and it can be dangerous if your medications interact with each other. Make sure that your doctor–all your doctors–know what drugs you're taking, including over-the-counter medications, herbs, vitamins, and other supplements.

Your Pharmacist: Your New Best Friend

If you're used to filling your prescriptions at some faceless, nameless chain and never seeing the same pharmacist twice, and/or never have more than a one-sentence con-versation with the pharmacist, consider switching. Here's why.

A good pharmacist is much more than a pill filler. He or she should also be tracking your medications via a computerized program that spits out warnings about drug interactions, and notices if you change to a different medication or start a new drug. The pharmacist can also provide counseling; patiently answer your questions about possible interactions with over-the-counter drugs, supplements, herbs, or vitamins; and provide advice and recommendations on diabetes products, including supplies.

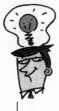

Sugar Sense _____

Always carry your pharmacy's fax and phone number with you when you go to the doctor and when you travel. That way, your doctor's office can fax or phone in your prescription so that it's ready when you arrive (no waiting). When you're traveling, an out-of-town pharmacy can contact your pharmacist for prescription information if necessary.

Online Drugs—Not a Good Idea

If you're like many Americans with a chronic illness, you might be considering ordering your drugs through an online pharmacy or even driving to Canada or Mexico to buy them so that you can save money. We don't think that's such a good idea, except under certain circumstances (which we tell you about later).

For one, it's illegal. For another, it's incredibly dangerous. In the summer of 2003, the U.S. Food and Drug Administration conducted a check of medications coming into the country from other countries. Nearly 90 percent of imported drugs checked contained medications that were not approved for use in the United States. Some of the drugs had been withdrawn from the U.S. market for safety reasons. Others were inappropriately packed in baggies, tissue paper, or envelopes—sometimes arriving crushed and broken. Most often, the drugs had inadequate labeling and instructions for safe and proper use. Sometimes the labeling wasn't in English and other times basic critical information, such as proper dosing, was missing.

In fact, the World Health Organization (WHO) estimates that 5 to 8 percent of all pharmaceutical products are counterfeit, with that figure reaching 70 percent in some parts of the world.

Often, online pharmacies tell you that it's *not* illegal to import drugs because the FDA has a "personal use" exemption. However, that exemption exists only in certain cases where a patient has a very serious condition for which no effective treatment is available in the United States. It certainly doesn't cover importing drugs such as oral diabetes medications or insulin.

Buying Online Safely

However, if you can't resist the prices or otherwise enjoy the convenience of online pharmacies, make sure you follow these tips to ensure that your pharmacy is legitimate and the medication you receive is safe:

- Make sure that your drug site is certified through the National Association of Boards of Pharmacies' (NABP) Verified Internet Pharmacy Practice Sites (VIPPS) program. You can get a list of VIPPS-approved pharmacies by going to http://www.nabp.net or calling 847-698-6227.

- Make sure that the site requires that you provide a bonafide prescription from a physician or other licensed healthcare provider. Keep away from any site that just has you complete a form to get the drugs.

- Make sure that the site provides you with direct access (phone and e-mail) to a registered pharmacist.

What's Your Problem?

Before we describe the five classes of drugs, let's discuss some general rules about how to decide which pill(s) to use. There are four things your doctor will probably consider when deciding this question.

- How effective is it? What is the best response you can expect if you take this pill? It turns out that all five classes of the oral drugs are pretty much equally effective.

- What are the side effects? Remember, no drug is entirely free of risk.

- How easy is it to take the medication? This affects how *compliant* you are in taking the drug. For instance, popping a pill once a day is easier than having to do it two or three times a day. And taking pills is certainly easier than injecting insulin.

- How much does the medication cost? As you probably know, *generic* drugs are much less expensive than name-brand drugs, which are still covered under exclusive patents.

MedLingo

A **generic** drug is one that has the same active ingredients as the branded drug, but is no longer protected by a patent. Thus, it can be produced by any drug company without paying royalties to the original developer of the drug, which means that the generic version is usually much less expensive than its branded cousin.

Your doctor will consider several things as he or she determines the right medication (or medications) for you:

MedLingo

Your body **metabolizes** a drug by breaking it down into its key components (usually in the liver) and then clearing the remainder of the drug and any resulting chemicals from your body, usually through your kidney (urine) and sometimes through the intestines (stool).

◆ Do you have any allergies to any medication? For instance, if you're allergic to sulfa antibiotics, you probably can't take any of the sulfonylurea medications (described later in this chapter).

◆ Are you overweight? Some medications can result in weight gain.

◆ Do you have kidney or liver damage? If so, it could affect how well your body is able to *metabolize*, or break down, the drug.

◆ What other drugs are you taking? Some might have dangerous interactions with oral diabetes medications.

Your doctor should take all of these issues into account when deciding which medication(s) to prescribe. Your doctor should also make sure that you understand the potential side effects of any new prescribed drugs.

However, it's just as important that you make sure your doctor has all the information he or she needs about your medical condition and lifestyle to make the appropriate decision, and that you get all your questions about the medications answered before you leave.

Sing a Song of Sulfonylureas

Sulfonylureas (pronounced SUL-fah-nil-YOO-ree-ahs) are the oldest class of oral diabetes drugs available, dating back to World War II. In fact, until 1996, they were all we had besides insulin to treat diabetes.

Sugar Sense

Always take your sulfonylurea medication at the same time every day.

They owe their discovery to observant researchers who were testing a new antibiotic sulfa drug in dogs. The researchers noticed that some of the dogs getting the drug died from hypoglycemia. Something about the drug was lowering their blood sugar levels. After much more research, bingo! The first noninjectable drug to treat diabetes was offered on the market in 1954.

Having been on the market for half a century, many different first- and second-generation sulfonylureas are available. Each of the SUs (as they're abbreviated) work in the same way: they kick your pancreas's insulin-making ability up a notch so that it makes more insulin, which helps lower blood glucose levels. However, this medication is only effective if your pancreas is still making *some* insulin.

The Downside

Sulfonylureas generally have some not-so-great side effects: weight gain (making your own efforts to *lose* weight more difficult) and hypoglycemia.

In addition, if you have significant kidney disease, only two of the sulfonylureas are safe (tolbutamide and glipizide).

> **Warning**
>
> All sulfonylureas can cause low blood glucose, particularly in the elderly, those with kidney problems, and those who don't adhere to a regular meal schedule. If you're taking one of these drugs, make sure to carry some kind of high-glucose snack or drink with you and remain aware of the early signs of hypoglycemia (more on hypoglycemia in Chapter 8).

When and How to Take

Today, you have a variety of sulfonylureas from which to choose. Which one you take depends on your doctor, your health insurance, and your individual medical condition. As of mid-2005, the FDA has approved the following sulfonylureas for marketing in the United States: Amaryl (glimepiride), DiaBeta (glyburide), Diabinese (chlorpropamide), acetohexamide (generic only), Glucotrol and Glucotrol XL (glipizide), Glynase PresTab and Micronase (glyburide), Orinase (tolbutamide), and Tolinase (tolazamide). All except Amaryl are also available in generic formulations, which makes them less expensive. In addition, Glucotrol XL and Amaryl offer a once-daily dosing.

Although all work similarly and have similar side effects, there are some subtle differences. For instance, Orinase, a short-acting formulation, might be best for the elderly and people with liver or kidney disease whose bodies don't metabolize drugs well. But, it has to be taken three times a day.

> **Bet You Didn't Know**
>
> About 15 percent of people who take Diabinese or its generic component will flush bright red in the face when they drink alcohol. Diabinese is the only SU that does this, however. So, if you get this reaction to this drug, either don't drink, or ask your doctor to give you another SU.

You usually take sulfonylureas before meals to avoid the hypoglycemia that might occur if you miss a meal. Glucotrol is usually more effective when taken 30 minutes before a meal; on the other hand, you can take Glucotrol XL *with* food. Diabinese is the longest-acting drug in the class, so you can get by on just one pill a day—a plus for anyone who hates taking pills. However, it's also the most likely to cause hypoglycemia. Most of the other types should be taken once or twice a day, depending on the dose.

The Big Deal About Biguanides

The class of drugs known as the biguanides (pronounced by-GWAN-ides) is relatively new in the United States. However, the most commonly prescribed biguanide, metformin, has been available for decades overseas. We didn't get it until 1995 because of the bad reputation of another drug in this class, phenformin.

Phenformin was available in the United States in the early 1970s, but was pulled off the market in 1976 because of a severe side-effect called *lactic acidosis*. This potentially fatal condition occurs when lactic acid, a byproduct of the transformation of glucose into energy, builds up in the body.

> **MedLingo**
>
> An **insulin sensitizer** improves how your body responds to insulin by increasing its effect both on putting glucose into muscle and fat cells and limiting the amount of glucose the liver releases.

No one is quite sure how metformin works, although we do know that it doesn't have anything to do with insulin secretion. Its main effect is to reduce the amount of glucose the liver produces when it senses insulin. It also helps insulin push glucose into muscle cells. Therefore, it is known as an *insulin sensitizer*.

How Good Is It?

Before we consider the side effects of metformin, we should mention a few positives. For one, instead of making you *gain* weight, it can help you lose weight initially (or, at the very least, not *gain* weight) by suppressing your appetite. Also, because metformin doesn't affect the amount of insulin your pancreas releases, it doesn't cause hypoglycemia. (But if it's added to a sulfonylurea or insulin, as it often is, you can wind up with low blood sugar). There's also some evidence that people with diabetes who take metformin are less likely to suffer heart attacks.

> **Bet You Didn't Know**
>
> Metformin is actually derived from the French lilac, which has been used as an herbal remedy for diabetes for hundreds of years.

One study looking at the ability of metformin to reduce long-term complications from diabetes found that overweight people taking the drug were 32 percent less likely to have any diabetes-related complications, 42 percent less likely to die from a diabetes-related cause, and 36 percent less likely to die overall during the study time than those receiving conventional diet therapy or treatment with an SU.

The Downside

Of course, there's always a downside. Metformin's side effects include gastrointestinal (GI) distress, such as bloating, abdominal pain, nausea, and diarrhea. This affects up to half of all people taking the drug. You might also notice a tinny or metallic taste in your mouth. You can minimize these side effects, however, by starting on small doses and gradually increasing the dose and also by taking the metformin when you eat. The gastrointestinal symptoms usually improve and often disappear in a week or two.

If your doctor increases your dose, however, you might find a temporary return of the GI symptoms. About 15 to 20 percent of people with diabetes can't tolerate metformin because of these symptoms, and some can handle only small doses.

There are also some reasons why you shouldn't use metformin. These are related to a very slight risk for lactic acidosis, the problem that got its cousin kicked off the market in the 1970s. As mentioned earlier, in lactic acidosis, the balance between acids and bases in your body gets out of whack, which can cause a lot of trouble. If you have any of the following, you have a higher risk for lactic acidosis and probably won't be started on metformin:

- **Kidney disease:** Because only the kidneys can eliminate metformin, if your kidneys aren't working properly, metformin reaches higher-than-normal levels in your blood stream.

- **Liver disease:** Because the liver metabolizes lactic acid, if your liver is not working properly, it can accumulate in the bloodstream.

- **Alcoholism:** When your liver is busy metabolizing high amounts of alcohol, lactic acid tends to accumulate in the bloodstream (although moderate intake of alcohol is not such a problem).

- **Heart failure:** If you have *congestive heart failure*, you might not have enough oxygen

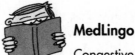

MedLingo

Congestive heart failure is a condition in which the heart doesn't pump enough blood.

going to your tissues. This lack of oxygen makes it more likely that lactic acidosis will result, even without adding a drug like metformin.

◆ **Over 80 years old:** As you age, your kidney function decreases. By the time you're 80 or older, your kidneys might not work well enough to properly eliminate metformin.

Which One and How to Take

Currently, metformin, marketed as Glucophage, is the only biguanide on the market. It comes in two formulations: regular, which must be taken two to three times a day with meals, and long-acting (Glucophage XR), which can be taken once a day with a meal. Only Glucophage is available in a generic form.

Going with the Alpha-Glucosidase Inhibitors (AGI)

This class of drugs, pronounced *AL-fa gloo-KOS-ih-dayss in-HIB-it-ers*, was introduced in 1986. They work very differently from the other two classes of drugs. Instead of affecting the way your body makes or responds to insulin, they slow the breakdown of carbohydrates in the small intestine after you eat. This delays your body's absorption of glucose, thus flattening out the post-meal blood sugar spikes.

How Good Are They?

When compared directly to an SU or metformin, they are a little less effective. Having said that, they are a great option if you're prone to high blood glucose levels after eating. On their own, they also won't put you at risk for hypoglycemia. An added bonus is that AGIs won't lead to weight gain.

The Downside

AGIs can cause gas, bloating, diarrhea, and abdominal discomfort from all those undigested carbohydrates hanging out in your intestines. Sometimes the side effects are bad enough that some people stop taking them. Still, these symptoms usually improve in a few weeks. So talk to your doctor about how you can minimize these side effects, such as starting with a smaller dose and gradually increasing it.

You probably also shouldn't take an AGI if you have gastrointestinal problems such as inflammatory bowel disease.

Which One and How to Take

Currently, there are two AGIs approved for sale in the United States: Precose (acarbose) and Glyset (miglitol). Because they slow the absorption of carbohydrates, each should be taken three times a day with the very first bite of food, although your doctor might have you take them less often in the beginning until your body gets used to their effects.

CAUTION   Warning

If you're taking AGIs along with an SU or insulin and you develop hypogly-cemia, make sure that you take a glucose tablet to raise your glucose levels. A carbo-hydrate-containing food or drink won't work fast enough because the AGI slows the absorption of the carbohydrate. It turns out that AGIs do not affect the breakdown of the carbohydrate in milk, however, so you can also use milk to treat low blood sugar if you're taking an AGI.

Bouncing Back from Adversity: Thiazolidinediones (TZD)

This class of drugs, pronounced *THIGH-ah-ZO-li-deen-DYE-owns*, (sometimes called glitazones for short) got off to a bad start when they were first introduced in 1997. The first drug in the class, called Rezulin, was pulled off the market in 2000 when it was found to cause severe liver damage in a few patients. However, two other drugs in this class, Avandia (rosiglitazone) and Actos (pioglitazone), each of which have been on the market since 1999, don't seem to have the same problem.

We're not quite sure exactly how these drugs work (this is more common than you'd think with many medications), but the end result is that they change the makeup of genes that regulate how your body metabolizes carbohydrates and fats. This, in turn, helps your muscles take in more glucose, thus decreasing insulin resistance and, of course, blood glucose levels. These drugs also reduce the amount of glucose your liver produces to some extent.

Bet You Didn't Know

Thiazolidinediones have a major effect on muscle and a minor effect on the liver, while metformin is just the opposite, it has a major effect on the liver and a minor effect on muscle.

An Added Bonus

TZDs might have another effect on the pancreas, however. Remember when we said earlier that the pancreas produces less insulin over time regardless of your treatment? People who take TZDs might be an important exception to this.

Early studies suggest that TZD might slow the eventual weakening of the pancreas. If true, this could enable you to stay on oral medications longer. Larger studies are now ongoing.

There's another potential advantage to TZDs. They increase the HDL (good) cholesterol, which usually starts out low in people with type 2 diabetes. However, they have a more complicated effect on LDL (bad) cholesterol.

To understand this effect, you need to know that cholesterol is carried around in the blood by certain proteins. Smaller, denser proteins carrying LDLs cause damage to the blood vessels while larger, less heavy ones don't. TZDs help by making these proteins lighter and more buoyant. So, although TZDs increase the amount of these proteins, thus increasing the levels of LDL cholesterol, they also make them less dangerous by changing their size.

Finally, TZDs can also lower blood pressure just a bit. All of these effects, along with the decrease in insulin resistance, should lower your risk for heart disease.

Several large studies are currently underway to test this theory. Unfortunately, it will be years before we have definitive results.

The Downside

You knew that the TZDs were sounding too good to be true, didn't you? As with every drug, there's always a downside. A minor one is that it can take up to a month to begin to see an effect, and up to four months to see the maximum effect.

A greater negative is that they can cause weight gain, even more than the SUs. So if you take a TZD, you need to be more careful with your diet.

They can also cause swelling of the legs in about 10 to 15 percent of patients, a side effect that is generally worse if you're also taking insulin. If you have congestive heart failure, you definitely should not take TZDs.

One final downside is that they are the most expensive class of oral drugs for diabetes.

Bet You Didn't Know

Be careful if you're a premenopausal woman taking a TZD. They may make birth-control pills less effective and trigger ovulation if you've stopped ovulating. Thus, if you haven't actually reached menopause (defined as 12 months since your last period), are on the pill, and don't want to get pregnant, make sure that you use another form of birth control while taking a TZD. (Metformin can also trigger ovulation, but it has no affect on birth control pills.)

Which One and How to Take

The two TZDs currently on the market, Avandia (rosiglitazone) and Actos (pioglitazone), are each taken once or twice a day. There is really only one difference between them: Pioglitazone lowers the levels of triglycerides, common in people with type 2 diabetes, whereas rosiglitazone doesn't seem to have any affect on triglyceride levels.

Messing with Meglitinides

You might hear this last class of drugs referred to as "non-SU secretagogues." This term refers to the fact that these drugs make the pancreas put out, or *secrete*, more insulin. They work similarly to the sulfonylureas, but tend to stimulate beta cells in short bursts, rather than over longer periods of time. Also, they increase insulin secretion only when blood sugar is high, not when it's normal, and certainly not when it's low. This reduces the risk of hypoglycemia.

You take meglitinides before meals. They're also good for people with irregular meal schedules. SUs can cause hypoglycemia if you miss a meal after taking one, but meglitinides increase the production of insulin only after you eat and blood sugar levels start to rise. So if you miss a meal, there's no increased insulin release and no hypoglycemia.

Two meglitinides are currently on the market: Prandin (repaglinide) and Starlix (nateglinide).

How Good Are They?

Meglitinides carry only a slight risk for hypoglycemia, but they can result in some weight gain, although less than SUs.

And there is kind of a big downside. They have to be taken more frequently than other medications, meaning before each meal, even before a large snack.

Choosing the Right Drug

If you think you're confused by now, just consider how your doctor feels. You're reading only a few pages about each drug; your doctor is exposed to numerous studies, presentations, and education about all these drugs—which is all designed by the drug manufacturers to get him or her to prescribe their particular drug to you. So how does your doctor choose, particularly given that most of the oral medications are equally effective in controlling diabetes?

They generally start with what's known as a *first-line treatment.* This is a drug that has been shown to be relatively safe and effective with few side effects. When it comes to oral diabetes medications for people who are overweight, that drug is often metformin.

If metformin is *contraindicated* or if you can't take it because of gastrointestinal side effects, an SU is usually the second choice. An SU may be the first choice of many doctors anyway because it is just as effective as metformin and a little cheaper.

On the other hand, because TZDs are designed to specifically treat insulin resistance and have the potential to improve blood vessel disease and perhaps preserve beta cell function, some doctors use a drug from this class as a first-line treatment.

MedLingo

First-line treatments are those drugs typically used first to treat a condition or disease because of their history of safety and effectiveness.

A drug is **contraindicated** if you have some medical conditions that might increase its negative side effects or cause other potential problems.

Combining Pills

If the first medication doesn't control your blood sugar well enough, most doctors will add a second drug from a different class. Because drugs in each class work via different mechanisms, it's not surprising that two will often be more effective than one.

If two don't do the job, your doctor might either add a third, or start you on insulin. Usually, in this case, you start taking insulin only at bedtime (more on that in the next chapter) and continue taking the oral medications you've been taking.

If your doctor starts you on three medications and they still don't do the job, then you're sure to be started on insulin, possibly even more than one injection.

Two Pills in One

Several pharmaceutical companies make oral diabetes medications that contain two medications, each from a different class. These can be helpful because many people with diabetes have to take several pills a day, a combination tablet cuts that number somewhat.

The combination tablets currently available are Glucovance (glyburide/metformin), Metaglip (glipizide/metformin), and Avandamet (Avandia/metformin). If you have a co-pay for your medication, the combination pills might save you some money. On the other hand, none are generic, so it might cost more to take a single combination pill than two generic pills. Check the prices!

The Least You Need to Know

♦ There are five classes of oral diabetes medications.

♦ Each oral medication works in a unique way, and each has its own benefits and downsides.

♦ Your doctor might put you on more than one oral diabetes drug, or might eventually combine oral medication with insulin.

♦ Make sure you take your medicine as directed.

♦ Even if you're on medication, you still need to maintain your diet and exercise regimen.

Beyond the Pills: Insulin

In This Chapter

- ◆ Understanding insulin
- ◆ Injecting insulin
- ◆ The various types of insulin
- ◆ Intensive insulin therapy
- ◆ Hypoglycemia

If you're reading this chapter, your doctor either just told you it was time to move to insulin, or you've been taking insulin for some time and want to know more about it. You've come to the right place.

First, you should not feel like you failed or did something wrong because your doctor is putting you on insulin. Even people whose HbA1c levels never rise above 6 percent, whose body weight remains perfect, and who exercise an hour every day may eventually need insulin. It just means that the beta cells in your pancreas have simply run out of steam. It's time to step in with all that modern medicine can provide.

Consider this chapter as your roadmap to the world of insulin. From the best needles and syringes to use, to the best insulin for *you*—you should be able to find your answers here.

Just What the Heck Is Insulin (and Why Doesn't It Come in a Pill?)

It's a modern medical miracle, that's what it is. Insulin was discovered over 80 years ago and earned its discoverers Nobel prizes. Think about *that* every time you prepare to draw up a dose.

Also consider yourself lucky to be living in the twenty-first century. Back in the early part of the last century, insulin was produced from pig and cow pancreases. This resulted in quite a few allergic reactions, which could make insulin very unpleasant to take. Rarely, it led to a certain kind of a reaction that made the insulin nearly worthless.

In the middle of the century, stricter manufacturing processes did away with the worst of the allergic reactions. Now the development of *recombinant human insulin* has made the insulin used today extremely pure and allergic reactions very rare.

A Bit of Chemistry

Two things to remember: Insulin is a protein, and all proteins are made out of long chains of building blocks called *amino acids*.

Today, we use genetic engineering to turn bacteria into little insulin-making factories, churning out enormous amounts of human insulin identical to that which your body produces.

MedLingo

Recombinant human insulin uses genetic engineering to turn bacteria into little insulin-producing factories. **Amino acids** are the building blocks of proteins. A few of the amino acids in the **insulin analogs** are changed by genetic engineering to change the way your body absorbs insulin.

But genetic engineering can also tell the bacteria to switch a few amino acids around or to add one or two extra to produce *insulin analogs*. Insulin analogs work just like human insulin, but they simply change the rate at which your body absorbs insulin.

Today, four analogs are available in the United States. Humalog (lispro), NovoLog (aspart), and Apidra (glulisine) speed up the insulin-absorbing process, while the fourth, Lantus (glargine), markedly slows it down. The analogs make insulin much more convenient to use because they better mimic your body's natural cycle of insulin production.

> **Bet You Didn't Know**
>
> The United States phased out all beef-based insulin products years ago; now it's doing the same with pork insulins. Today, if you're newly diagnosed with diabetes and put on insulin, you take either an analog or human insulin. Pork insulin is still made and used by some people who have been taking it for years, but it will soon be a memory like the Model T and wired telephones.

Why the Needles?

You'd think that if we can send a human being to the moon (several times), take pictures of Mars, and invent TiVo, we could figure out how to get insulin into a pill. Trust us, it's easier to send someone to the moon.

As we noted earlier, insulin is a protein. And just like the protein in the swordfish you had for dinner last night, your body loves to break it down in your intestines so that it can absorb the amino-acid building blocks.

So if you took insulin by mouth, when it passed through your digestive system it would be toast (well, actually, just a bunch of amino acids) by the time it got to your blood system. It certainly wouldn't work as insulin any more. Injecting it directly into your body ensures that it passes quickly into your bloodstream where it works the way it's supposed to.

Don't worry; as you read later on, researchers are investigating some pretty cool new delivery methods for insulin, ranging from insulin patches to inhaled insulin, even—gasp!—an insulin pill. You can read more about the new insulins in Chapter 22.

So How Much Do I Need?

That depends on many factors. You might need insulin only once a day, maybe at night, and might be able to control your blood sugar levels the rest of the time with oral medications.

Or you might need to be on a mixture of different types of insulin injected before breakfast and before supper. Or you might inject one type before each meal and another type at bedtime. You might even inject a mixture before breakfast, another type before supper, and a third type before bed.

It's up to you and your doctor to work together to find the combination that works best.

There are nearly as many options when it comes to the dosing. How much insulin you take depends on your weight, activity level, diet, the blood sugar goals you and your doctor set, and how your body responds to insulin.

Insulin works differently in each person; what works great for your neighbor might not be the best option for you. Plus, insulin can even work differently in your body from day to day—depending on what's going on in your life. Menstruation, vacations, stress, differences in what you eat from day to day—these can all affect the amount you need.

Because the amount you need is not a static amount, it's a good idea to make sure your doctor or diabetes educator trains you to adjust your insulin doses based on your individual circumstances at any given time.

It all sounds rather complicated, but if you work closely with your doctor, it's not as tough as it seems. The ultimate goal is to mimic the natural action of a healthy pancreas, providing just enough insulin to balance your blood sugar, but not so much to send you into hypoglycemia. (There's more about hypoglycemia, or low blood sugar, at the end of this chapter.)

What's My Dose?

In the United States, insulin is marketed in 10-ml vials at a concentration of 10 units (usually abbreviated as U) per milliliter. The dose is given in units, so, for instance, you might be asked to take 10 U before breakfast.

> **CAUTION**
>
> **Warning**
>
> Don't take a warm shower (or bath) for one to two hours after taking insulin. The warm water increases blood flow to your skin, causing insulin to be absorbed faster, which could cause hypoglycemia.

Fortunately, you won't have to do any calculations to get that amount. The syringe you use has the number of units marked right on it. You simply draw up the fluid from the vial to the 10 marked on the syringe. This syringe is called a U-100 syringe (to be used with U-100 insulin) and holds up to 1 ml. This means that each syringe, if full, holds 100 units.

Other countries, however, have other concentrations, usually U-40 (which is a more diluted concentration). But they also have U-40 syringes with the number of units marked right on the syringe.

Thus, it's very important to use only U-100 syringes with U-100 insulin and U-40 syringes with U-40 insulin. Otherwise, you'll get the wrong amount of insulin. If you never buy insulin in another country, just ignore all of this. If you do buy U-40 insulin in another country, make sure that you also get U-40 syringes. If not, you'll be in big trouble.

Getting Over Needle Phobia

Let's face it, no one likes needles (except maybe the needle manufacturers). But the needles on insulin syringes are very small, designed to be as pain free as possible. Plus, the tip is very, very sharp. The needle is also coated with silicone, a slippery substance that helps it slip right into your skin, almost without you noticing it.

Today, some insulins also come in pens. They look like regular pens, but instead of an ink-filled cartridge, they're filled with insulin. There's still a tiny needle on the end of the pen, but there's no filling of syringes and no really obvious needle. You just turn a dial to pick the dose of insulin you want, press a plunger on the end, and bingo! You've got your injection.

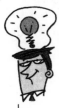

Sugar Sense

Almost anyone can get over the fear of sticking him or herself. However, if you're still having a bit of trouble giving yourself a shot, try these techniques:

◆ Set a reward for yourself after every injection. It could be watching a favorite TV show, savoring a bite of chocolate (just one bite), or curling up with a good book.

◆ Use visual imagery to relax yourself. Close your eyes and picture yourself in a place that makes you happy and relaxed. When you feel your breathing and heartbeat slow down, open your eyes and give yourself the injection.

◆ Create a special place in your home where you always give yourself your injections. Put a picture of a loved one there to remind you of why this is so important, some scented potpourri to make it a more pleasant place, all your supplies, and a trashcan.

You can also skip needles altogether. A device called an insulin jet injector uses high-pressure air to push a fine spray of insulin through your skin. Available brands include AdvantaJet, Medi-ject, and Injex. Some studies even suggest that the devices, which deliver insulin in a fine stream, allow the hormone to immediately enter tiny blood vessels, called capillaries, and be absorbed more quickly into your bloodstream. With the development of analog insulins, however, this quick absorption isn't as important as it used to be.

Additionally, subcutaneous infusion sets, also called insulin infusers, provide another alternative. You insert a *catheter* (a thin, flexible tube) into the tissue just beneath your skin and tape the entrance to the catheter to your abdomen. The tube remains in place for several days and you inject insulin into the infuser entrance instead of through your skin. Finally, you can even buy a device that hooks onto the syringe and pushes the needle into your skin with a quick, dart-like motion, so you don't have to do it.

Preparing to Stick

Certainly, if your doctor told you that you need to take insulin, you've had a lesson in injecting yourself. Probably flew in one ear and out the other, right? So here's how it's done:

1. Thoroughly wash your hands.

2. Remove the cap from a new bottle of insulin. If you're using a cloudy preparation (more on that later), roll the bottle between the palms of your hands to mix. Make sure the cloudy sediment at the bottom of the bottle (which is the insulin) mixes well with the rest of the fluid.

3. Wipe the rubber stopper and the top of the bottle with an alcohol wipe or cotton moistened with alcohol.

4. Holding the bottle in an upright position on a tabletop or other firm surface, insert the needle through the center of the rubber stopper.

5. Turn the bottle upside down and make sure that the needle tip is covered with insulin.

6. Pull back on the plunger of the syringe to your prescribed dose (which is written on the syringe), and then push it up again. Repeat this two or three times to eliminate air bubbles in the syringe. Air bubbles won't hurt you, but they will prevent you from drawing an accurate dose of insulin into the syringe.

7. Pull back on the plunger very slowly to your prescribed dose.

8. Pull the needle out of the bottle, taking care not to touch it. After injecting yourself, dispose of the syringe in a safe manner.

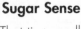

Sugar Sense _____

That tiny needle might look innocuous, but it's considered medical waste and needs to be disposed of appropriately. You need some equipment: a tool that clips, catches, and contains the needle and an opaque heavy-duty plastic bottle with a top or a plastic or metal box that you can close tightly. Don't use scissors; they could send the tip of the needle flying. When the box or bottle is full, check with your local waste authority as to the best way to dispose of it.

Avoiding That "Pin Cushion" Feeling

You don't just pick up a syringe filled with insulin and plunge it into yourself any ol' way. It's important to give yourself a *subcutaneous injection*, meaning an injection into the fat layer just below the skin. This differs from an *intramuscular injection*, which means injecting deeper into the muscle. Don't do that! If you do, the insulin will be absorbed too fast. Also avoid injecting close to blood vessels you can see through your skin.

MedLingo _____

A **subcutaneous injection** is an injection into the layer of fat just beneath the skin; an **intramuscular** injection is one that goes into a muscle. If you hit muscle, it will usually hurt more.

Choosing the Right Injection Site

The ideal injection sites are your abdomen, legs, arms, and buttocks. If you choose your abdomen, use the area about two inches below your belly button, anywhere between your hips. You can try the fleshy back part of your arm midway between your shoulder and elbow or the top of your thigh about six inches below your groin and above your knee. If you choose your butt, obviously you can only hit the part you can reach.

It really does matter *where* you inject, because insulin is absorbed differently depending on where the dose goes (except with Lantus insulin). So, ideally, you should pick one main area and stick to it (pun intended). The abdomen is the preferred spot.

That doesn't mean sticking yourself in the same spot every time. Instead, vary the location by about an inch each time, but keep using the same part of the body. Do it in an orderly fashion, not returning to the same injection site for at least a week. So, for instance, if you choose your abdomen, start near one hip and work your way across the abdomen to the other hip, and then go up an inch and start back.

CAUTION

Warning

Injecting into the same spot over and over again can lead to an accumulation of fat at that spot, making the absorption of insulin erratic (not constant from one day to the next).

Also, it's important to understand that if you exercise the place where you inject insulin (for example, injecting into your arm and then lifting weights), the insulin will be absorbed faster.

Making the Stick

When it's time to inject, and you've got just the right place in mind, here's how to do it:

1. Clean the injection site with an alcohol wipe or cotton moistened with alcohol.

2. If you're skinny (lucky you!) pinch or bunch up the skin with your whole hand to lift the fat from the muscle tissue below. If your flesh is firm but fat, spread the skin with your hand.

Sugar Sense

Is your insulin leaking from the injection site? You might be injecting it too quickly, releasing the skin before removing the needle, or inserting the needle at an incorrect angle, injecting the insulin just under your skin instead of into the fatty tissue below.

3. Holding your syringe like a pencil, touch the needle to your skin at a 90-degree angle (like an upside-down "T").

4. Insert the full length of the needle straight into your skin.

5. Inject the insulin at a steady rate, neither slow nor fast.

6. Remove the needle and press a cotton ball or alcohol wipe firmly on the injection site, holding it there for a few seconds. Do not rub.

Long, Short, Medium, Tall ... Picking the Right Insulin

The number of insulin types, as well as the names and choices among them, are enough to give you a migraine. There are five primary types: rapid-acting, short-acting, intermediate-acting, long-acting, and pre-mixed.

With each type, you want to know three things:

◆ Onset: This is how long it takes before the insulin hits your bloodstream and begins doing its job.

◆ Peak time: This is how long it takes after injection for the insulin to do its best job (peak) at lowering your blood sugar. One insulin, Lantus, is *peakless*, which, as you might suspect, means it doesn't have a peak. It has the same effect for about 24 hours after injection.

◆ Duration: This is how long the insulin keeps working in your body to lower blood glucose levels. After its peak effect, it gradually wears off until its effect is gone.

The following table summarizes the timing of insulin preparations. Note that the times have a broad range. This reflects two things: the tremendous variability between individuals and their reactions to insulin, and the difficulty in accurately measuring the timing of when insulin starts to work, has its peak effect, and how long it lasts.

That's why you have to work closely with your doctor. There are no easy rules that apply to everyone when it comes to adjusting insulin doses, although there are some important relationships between the types of insulin used, when it's injected, and when you should test your blood sugar that determines how to adjust insulin doses. We get to these later in the chapter.

MedLingo

Peakless insulin has a steady effect on blood sugar, without any highs or lows that could lead to hypoglycemia.

Insulin Preparations

Type (generic)	Brand name	Onset of action	Peak of action	Duration of action
Rapid-Acting	Humalog (lispro)	5-15 minutes	30-90 minutes	3-5 hours
	NovoLog (aspart)			
	Apidra (glulisine)			
Short-Acting (regular)	Humulin R	30-60 minutes	2-4 hours	4-6 hours
(also called ReliOn, but available only through Wal-Mart)	Novolin R			
Intermediate Acting	Humulin N Novolin N	About 3 hours	6-12 hours	8-24 hours
	Humulin L			
	Novolin L			
Intermediate and short-acting mixtures	Humulin mix 50/50	Depends on the individual mixture		
	Humulin mix 70/30			
Immediate/ regular)	Humalog mix 50/50			
	Novolin mix 70/30			
	Novolog mix 70/30			
Long-acting	Ultralente	4-8 hours	8-16 hours	36 hours
Lantus (glargine)	1 hour		None	24 hours

Rapid-Acting Insulin: Get Me My Insulin and Get It to Me Now!

Currently, three rapid-acting insulins are on the market, all insulin analogs: Humalog, NovoLog, and Apidra. As their name implies, rapid-acting insulins begin working right away, generally within 5 to 15 minutes of injection. That's why they're generally taken right before meals to help with the glucose spike that typically starts about 20 minutes after you start eating and can last three to four hours.

The analogs lower your blood sugar within about 45 minutes to two hours. And, as an added advantage, they only hang around a few hours, so they're less likely to lead to hypoglycemia. In fact, one study found that people using Humalog had 25 percent fewer episodes of serious hypoglycemia than those using regular insulin. (Serious hypoglycemia is defined as a situation where you are so out of it that you can't treat yourself, and someone has to help you.)

These rapid-acting insulins offer a flexibility previously unavailable to people with diabetes. In the past, to reduce glucose spikes after a meal, people with diabetes had to take the short-acting regular insulin 30 minutes before they began eating. Frankly, most people are just not that organized and life just doesn't run on such a strict schedule.

The analog insulins, however, can be injected just before you start to eat. They can even be taken right after a meal; so if you ate more or less than you expected, you can change your dose accordingly.

The biggest drawback? These insulin analogs (including the long-acting insulin Lantus) are considerably more expensive than human insulins.

> **Sugar Sense**
>
> Confused as to the difference between short-acting and rapid-acting? You're not alone. Put simply, the insulin analogues are called rapid acting, while regular insulin is called short-acting. Both have about the same time of duration once injection.

> **Warning**
>
> If you like to exercise within one to three hours of eating, make sure to take a lower dose of a rapid-acting insulin to avoid the risk of hypoglycemia. If you exercise later, you don't need to worry about changing your dose.

Short-Acting or Regular Insulin: Predictable and Boring, but Effective

The two most commonly used short-acting insulins in the United States are Eli Lilly's Humulin R and Novo Nordisk's Novolin R. Note the "R" after the name of the insulin; that's your clue that we're talking "regular" insulin here. Also note the manufacturers: Eli Lilly and Novo Nordisk dominate the insulin marketplace in this county, indeed, in the world.

Short-acting insulins, which are always clear (as are the rapid-acting insulins), generally begin working about 30 to 60 minutes after you take them, reach their peak action about two to four hours after injection, and keep working for about four to six hours. Like the rapid-acting insulins, they're injected before meals.

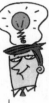

Sugar Sense _____

You don't just pick up a prescription of insulin and toss it in the back seat of your car. Insulin is a delicate hormone; it needs to be treated with respect. That means avoiding excessive heat (in the car, on your windowsill, or near the stove), shaking it *gently* when you're mixing it, and keeping it out of freezing temperatures. Although insulin stays fresh for weeks or even months at room temperature, if you buy a bunch at one time, keep it in the fridge just to be on the safe side.

Intermediate Acting Insulin: Not Too Hot, Not Too Cold

There are two forms of intermediate-acting insulin: NPH and Lente. NPH stands for the tongue-twisting Neutral Protamine Hagedorn. It has an extra protein added to it, the *protamine*, which slows down your body's absorption of insulin. The other type, Lente (L), is absorbed more slowly because of the size of the insulin crystal. Both are cloudy, which easily distinguishes them from short-acting insulins.

These insulins, which include the brands Humulin N and L, and Novolin N and L, start to work in about three hours, peak at around six to 12 hours, and keep working for 18 to 24 hours. You generally take this form of insulin in the morning to control your blood sugar in the afternoon or in the evening to control your blood sugar overnight.

> **Bet You Didn't Know**
>
> "Neutral Protamine Hagedorn" is named after the chemist who first joined insulin to protamine in the 1930s, Hans Christian Hagedorn, a Dane who also developed the first method for determining blood sugar.

Long-Acting Insulin: In for the Long Haul

The long-acting insulins are called *basal insulins* because they are designed to maintain a base level of insulin throughout the day and night. The first long-acting analog, Lantus (glargine) was approved for marketing in the United States in the Spring of 2001. After it is injected, Lantus insulin is slowly released into your bloodstream and is effective for about 24 hours. There is less overnight hypoglycemia with Lantus insulin compared to intermediate-acting insulins taken in the evening.

The other form of long-acting insulin, called Ultralente, has bigger crystals than Lente insulin, thus its absorption is even slower. Ultralente is effective for about 36 hours.

Something very important to keep in mind: Lantis is the only long-acting insulin that is clear (like the rapid- and short-acting insulins). The intermediate-acting insulins and the long-acting insulin, Ultralente, are cloudy. One more thing to remember: We talk later about mixing rapid- and short-acting insulins with the intermediate-acting insulins in the same syringe. Lantus inulin must be injected separately; it can't be mixed with other insulins.

Premixed Insulins: A Little of This; a Little of That

Premixed insulins, which are always cloudy, might be a good option if you're taking more than one kind but don't want to have to mix the two yourself. Premixed insulins come already mixed in the vial (duh!) so you simply draw them up in a syringe and inject them. They're also available in a pen form, which is a much easier form to carry around.

Most brands offer a 70 percent NPH and a 30 percent regular mixture, although one of the newest insulins on the market, Humalog Mix 75/25, contains 75 percent lispro protamine (in other words, lispro attached to protamine) and 25 percent rapid-acting lispro insulin. Not to be outdone, competitor Novo Nordisk has its own analog mixture of 70 percent aspart protamine and 30 percent rapid-acting aspart.

Note that we said that the premixed insulins "might be" a good option. They have one serious drawback. It can be difficult to maintain your blood sugars near normal throughout the day when using them. We explain why in a minute.

> **Bet You Didn't Know**
>
> People with diabetes who live in Arab deserts without refrigeration learn to bury their insulin in the sand to keep it cool.

The Insulin Bartender: Mixing Insulins

If you don't buy your insulins already premixed, you have to mix them yourself. Here's the drill:

1. Thoroughly wash your hands.

2. Roll the bottle of cloudy (intermediate-acting or long-acting) insulin between your hands to mix it. Clear (rapid- or short-acting insulin) doesn't need any mixing.

Warning _____

Remember: Lantus insulin is also a clear insulin, but it shouldn't be mixed with other insulins.

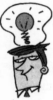

Sugar Sense _____

If mixing is just too cumbersome for you, ask a family member to do it for you. If someone is not available every time you need to mix and inject insulin, then either a family member or a nurse in your doctor's office can prepare a number of prefilled syringes for you.

3. Wipe the rubber stoppers and tops of both bottles with an alcohol wipe or cotton moistened with alcohol.

4. Holding the bottle of clear insulin in an upright position on a tabletop or other firm surface, insert the needle through the center of the rubber stopper.

5. Turn the bottle upside down and make sure the needle tip is covered with insulin.

6. Pull back on the plunger of the syringe to your prescribed dose of clear insulin, and then push it up again. Repeat this two or three times to eliminate air bubbles in the syringe.

7. Withdraw your prescribed dose of clear insulin from the bottle.

8. Pull the needle out of the bottle, taking care not to touch it.

9. Insert the needle into the bottle of cloudy insulin.

10. Turn the bottle upside down and pull back the plunger of your syringe very slowly to add the correct amount of cloudy insulin. Remember to take into account the amount of clear insulin already in the syringe. For example, if you have 10 units of clear insulin in the syringe and need to add 40 units of cloudy insulin, you must draw the plunger back to the 50-unit mark.

11. If you draw too much cloudy insulin into the syringe, throw the whole thing away and start over. Don't inject it back into the bottle; that will contaminate the cloudy insulin with the clear insulin. And don't try to "fix" your mistake by squirting some of the insulin out of the syringe. You will only to wind up with an inaccurate dose.

Understanding the Relationship Between Type and Timing of Insulin and Blood Sugar Levels

There are very important relationships between the types of insulin you use, when you inject them, and the timing of your glucose tests. Your doctor uses this relationship to make decisions about adjusting your insulin doses. This topic is covered in detail in Chapter 11, but before you leave this chapter, you need to know about this relationship.

People on insulin generally take their injections before meals or at bedtime (short- and rapid-acting insulin are taken only before meals). Glucose tests also need to be done before eating and before a bedtime snack. (The following table shows you when to test, depending on which type of insulin you're using.

The table also explains why it can be more difficult to get your blood sugars close to normal with premixed insulin. Suppose your tests show pretty normal glucose values before supper but high levels before lunch. Ideally, you'd increase your morning dose so that the short- or rapid-acting insulin can lower your blood glucose levels by the time you test before lunch. But if you do that using premixed insulin, the greater increase will be in the intermediate-acting insulin (because it makes up the bulk of the premixed insulin), which might make the before-supper glucose levels too low.

By mixing your insulin yourself, you can increase just the short- or rapid-acting insulin to take care of the high before-lunch values, without running the risk of too-low values before supper.

Sugar Sense

If you're taking insulin, you should eat a small bedtime snack before going to sleep to avoid low blood sugars overnight.

Injecting Insulin and Glucose Testing

Type of Insulin	When Injected	Glucose Test
Rapid* and short	Before breakfast	Before lunch
Intermediate	Before breakfast	Before supper
Rapid* and short	Before lunch	Before supper
Rapid* and short	Before supper	Before bedtime snack
Intermediate	Before supper or at bedtime	Before breakfast
Long	Any time	Before breakfast

*Some doctors may ask you to test one to two hours after eating if you use a rapid-acting insulin.

Now you're on the same page as your doctor. And with some instructions from your doctor, you might be able to adjust your own insulin doses!

Hold Me Tight! Intensive Insulin Therapy

Ever since the results of the Diabetes Control and Complications Trial (DCCT) were published in 1993, it's become clear that intensive (in other words, tight) control of blood sugar levels is the best way to prevent diabetes-related complications. What does this mean?

It means using insulin, diet, and exercise to mimic the blood sugar levels of a person without diabetes—no matter what you're doing. Because no one day is the same, this means being flexible with your daily insulin injections and doing an awful lot of blood glucose testing.

Intensive insulin therapy is provided in three primary ways. The first is called a *basal/bolus* regimen. You take three or more insulin injections—short- or rapid-acting insulin before meals and intermediate or longer-acting insulin before bed. Because you take the short- or rapid-acting insulin before meals and their effect wears off relatively soon, the timing of your meals can vary somewhat.

You can also obtain intensive insulin therapy with an insulin pump, which provides even more flexibility. They're expensive, though, and require some more work on your part. We'll talk more about pumps in Chapter 9.

You can also achieve tight control with a *mixed/split* regimen. In the mixed/split regimen, you take a mixture of intermediate-acting and either short- or rapid-acting insulin before breakfast (not premixed; you mix it). Then you take either the same mixture or just the short- or rapid-acting insulin before supper. Finally, you take intermediate-acting insulin at bedtime. The downside to this regimen is that your exercise and eating patterns must be pretty much the same from day to day; in other words, there's much less flexibility.

Tight insulin management isn't for everyone. It's probably not for you if you don't like to …

- Follow a fairly strict schedule of eating, exercising, injections, and so on.
- Closely track your blood sugar (which means testing a lot).
- Remain closely aware of how much you exercise.
- Follow a meal plan pretty closely.

There are also some downsides to intensive insulin therapy, namely, increased risk of hypoglycemia and weight gain. "What?" you're screaming, "weight gain?" Well, it's ironic, but better control of your blood sugar levels means more blood sugar is getting into your cells. If you're not using up that energy through daily living and exercise, it will be converted into fat. Sorry about that. Maybe you need to review parts of Chapter 6.

How Low Can You Go? Avoiding and Coping with Hypoglycemia

If you're taking insulin, only one thing is standing between you and a lifetime of normal blood glucose levels—hypoglycemia, or low blood sugar. We've talked a lot about this throughout this and other chapters. Now it's time to focus a bit more on it.

Hypoglycemia is nothing to be taken lightly; it's a matter of considerable concern for people with diabetes and can even be fatal.

The crux of hypoglycemia lies with your brain's need for a continual supply of blood sugar, which it gets from your blood. When blood glucose levels are normal or even high, the brain is doing just fine and getting all that it needs. Let your levels fall below normal, however, and your brain begins to gasp for glucose. It literally begins starving. Hence the shakiness, headache, anxiety, and confusion that are the hallmarks of hypoglycemia. Other symptoms include sweating, hunger, and itching or burning of your skin.

The scary thing about hypoglycemia is that it can come on very quickly, and because one of the effects is confusion, you may not recognize it in yourself. That's why it's so important to always wear a MedicAlert bracelet that lets people know you have diabetes. It's also important to let people you see every day know about your condition, just in case something happens. In one instance, a first-grade teacher who had a severe hypoglycemic reaction lucked out when his kids noticed him behaving strangely and called for help.

Most important is, don't ignore the early signs of hypoglycemia: that shakiness and lightheadedness. It isn't going to go away; it will only get worse.

Carbs Are Your Friends

Luckily, the treatment for hypoglycemia is fairly simple and works pretty quickly: sugar. You need to get some carbohydrate—the purer the better—into your system as quickly as possible.

Most people with diabetes, particularly those who take insulin or certain oral medications, always carry some form of carbohydrate with them, whether it's juice, crackers, milk, or glucose tablets. An initial dose of about 20 grams of carbs should be enough to get you feeling better; follow that every 15 to 20 minutes if your symptoms haven't improved. After your levels rise, have a bit more to eat, even a full meal.

> **Sugar Sense**
>
> You may feel panicky if you have hypoglycemia and begin eating very fast to halt the feeling. Slow down. It can take 10 to 15 minutes for the glucose from carbohydrates to get into your bloodstream. But if you keep eating, you're going to tip the balance in the other direction and wind up with hyperglycemia.

Good options for treating hypoglycemia include the following:

- A handful of raisins
- A few Lifesavers or mints (*not* sugar free!)
- 4 to 6 ounces of orange juice or regular soda
- $1/2$ cup of skim milk

If you're prone to severe hypoglycemia and find yourself unable to swallow anything, your doctor may prescribe an injectable form of the hormone glucagon, which stimulates your liver to release glucose. Make sure that someone in your family and/or workplace knows how to administer the injection and where you keep the supplies. You can store it in the refrigerator for years so that it's available when you need it.

Finally, make sure to track your hypoglycemic episodes, including their severity, what you'd eaten in the few hours before them, which insulin you'd taken, and what you were doing. All of this will help your doctor fine-tune your regimen to avoid episodes in the future.

The Least You Need to Know

- Using insulin doesn't mean that you've failed at managing your diabetes.

- There are several different types of insulin; which ones you take and how often will depend on your individual medical condition, your lifestyle, and other factors that your doctor will consider.

- Needles are the most common delivery system for insulin, but pens and jet injectors are also available.

- There are specific steps to follow when filling a syringe with insulin and giving yourself an injection.

- Hypoglycemia is always a potential problem when you take insulin. Be prepared to deal with it.

Chapter 9

All Insulin, All the Time: External Insulin Pumps

In This Chapter

- All about insulin pumps
- Are insulin pumps right for you?
- Daily life with an insulin pump

You say you're tired of shots and pills? Have we got good news for you. How about a device about the size of an iPod that you wear on your belt or hidden beneath a layer of clothing? It's a device that delivers a fast-acting insulin through a tiny plastic tube at a steady rate all day and night (thus providing the best basal insulin possible), and, with the press of a button, gives you an extra boost just before meals. It's an approach that mimics the way your body produced insulin before you got diabetes. Plus, there are no needles. No alcohol swabs. No fuss or mess.

Welcome to the wonderful world of the external insulin pump. For years, external insulin pumps were the domain of people with type 1 diabetes. Today, however, with greater control of blood sugar a priority in people with both types, they're gaining ground among those with type 2. This means that most of the research conducted so far on external insulin pumps has been done in people with type 1. A nitpicky point to be sure, but one we want you to be aware of.

The History of Insulin Pumps

Although they've been around for more than 20 years, insulin pumps, also called Continuous Subcutaneous Infusion of Insulin (CSII), are still fairly uncommon in the world of type 2 diabetes. Part of that is the expense (more about that later), and part of that is simply because doctors seem to associate the pumps more with type 1 diabetes than with type 2.

The first long-term study that compared the effectiveness of insulin pumps to daily multiple shots of insulin in people with type 2 diabetes showed some interesting results. The study, published in the September 2003 issue of the journal *Diabetes Care*, found that after three months, those taking insulin and those using the pump showed similar improvements in blood sugar levels. But—and here's the great news—nearly all those on the pump preferred it to daily injections. It was more convenient, easier to use, and provided more flexibility, they said.

Get Out Your Pocketbook

Pumps ain't cheap! They cost, on average, about $6,000, with about another $1,500 to $2,000 spent on supplies each year. Although many insurance companies will cover the cost, they usually don't cover the entire cost. If you have a deductible to meet or even just a 20 percent co-payment, you could be paying some fairly significant out-of-pocket costs.

The good news is that Medicare covers the cost of pumps if you meet certain criteria. That includes a low C-peptide level. What, you're asking, is a C-peptide and what does it have to do with my diabetes? C-peptide is a lab test that measures insulin production. Obviously, if you have type 1 diabetes, it's going to measure little or no production, a clear sign that an insulin pump is appropriate.

This measurement was instituted in 2000 when the Centers for Medicare and Medicaid (CMS) first approved coverage of the pumps. At that time, they wanted to make sure that only people who really had type 1 diabetes used the pumps.

In 2002, CMS modified that ruling to allow people with type 2 diabetes to receive coverage for the pumps. At the same time, the agency raised the cut-off point for the C-peptide level for those with type 2 by 10 percent. So make sure your doctor orders this test if you plan on using a pump.

Bet You Didn't Know

A survey of 12,525 members of the American Diabetes Association and the American Association of Diabetes Educators found that more than half of doctors and nurses with type 1 diabetes reported using insulin pumps rather than traditional syringe therapy, a pump rate nearly 10 times higher than that of the overall type 1 diabetes population. Obviously, medical professionals are pretty keen on pumps!

Pump Basics

Pumps provide a steady infusion of insulin throughout the day to maintain a basal rate of blood insulin. But when you need a bolus dose, such as when you eat, you just push a button one or two times and voilà! A burst of insulin is provided to manage your meal. Think how convenient that would be when you're eating out; you could adjust the size of the dose depending on what you order without fumbling with needles and alcohol wipes.

Navigating Your Way Around a Pump

Today, five pump manufacturers market their wares in the United States: Animas Corporation, Dana Diabecare USA, Deltec, Inc., Medtronic Mini-Med, and Nipro Diabetes Systems. All their pumps work similarly, although they get fancier and easier to use every year.

For instance, Animas's newest pump, the IR 1200, is waterproof at 12 feet for 24 hours and offers automatic carb calculations. Medtronic Mini-Med's pumps have alarms that warn you if the battery is getting low. They even come in cool colors like ice blue, purple, and slate gray.

There are three parts to an external insulin pump:

◆ **The pump:** Weighing in at about 14 ounces, these pager-size devices have a read-out display and operational buttons on the front of the device. They hook onto your belt or slip into a pocket.

◆ **The infusion set:** This consists of thin plastic tubing. One end is connected to the pump, while the other has a tiny needle or *cannula* (also called a catheter) with a tiny tapered tube on the end that is inserted into the layer of fat just beneath the skin on some part of your body, typically your abdomen. You change the site of the insertion about every two to three days. If you have two unexplained high glucose readings in a row, check the cannula. A blocked cannula is the most common problem. It this occurs, change the cannula.

◆ **The reservoir:** This is the insulin-filled cartridge or syringe contained within the device itself. It has to be refilled about every two or three days.

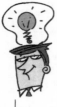

Sugar Sense

You don't just strap on a pump and hit the beach. Learning to use it properly and regulate the amount of insulin you need with the amount you give yourself takes time and practice. So sign up for a pump class. These three- to four-hour classes teach you everything you need to know about the care and feeding of your pump. Check with your local hospital or talk to your diabetes educator about a class near you. Some pump manufacturers even offer online courses!

Linking Monitoring and Infusion

In the past couple of years, several pump manufacturers have introduced new pump/monitor combinations. They use wireless technology to link the two together so that the glucose meter can send readings directly to the pump, reducing the risk of errors if you have to type in the numbers.

The Medtronic MiniMed Paradigm 512 Insulin Pump and Paradigm Link Blood Glucose Monitor go a step further. When the information from the glucose meter is transmitted, the pump considers the previous insulin dose, the amount of insulin still active in the body, the glucose level, and the amount of carbohydrates you're planning to eat (which you entered into the meter), and then determines the correct bolus, or dose, to be delivered.

The Paradigm 512 also transmits data directly to communications software on your computer, enabling you to easily track blood glucose levels.

The downside of these gadgets is that you still have to manually test your blood. But there's hope. Researchers are developing glucose meters that automatically test your blood sugar levels and send that information to the pump in an automated closed loop system with no finger sticks and no buttons to press.

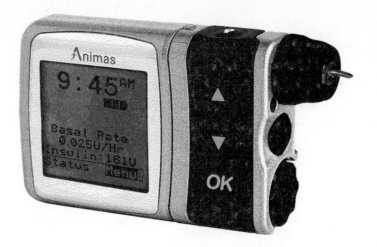

*Medtronic Paradigm 512
Insulin Pump and
Paradigm Link Monitor.*

What's the Best Insulin?

You can't use just any ol' insulin in a pump (although some people try). The best insulin, meaning the one least likely to clog the machine, is called buffered insulin. The three brands currently available in the United States are Velosulin CSII, which is a buffered regular, short-acting insulin, and Humalog (lispro) and NovoLog (aspart), which are both rapid-acting insulins. You don't need intermediate- or long-acting insulin, because the fast-acting insulins are delivered at a steady, slow trickle all the time.

Humalog has several advantages over Velosulin CSII when used in a pump. Studies find that it results in less severe and fewer cases of hypoglycemia with better control of blood sugars. Most likely, you can also expect the same from NovoLog.

Supplying Your Pump

Owning a pump is like owning a small puppy—you're constantly buying things for it. In addition to the regular diabetes supplies you still need to maintain (glucose meter, testing strips, syringes, needles, and so on), you also need to make sure you have the following:

- Extra reservoir
- Batteries for the pump
- Insertion device

- Alcohol swabs

- Tape and adhesives (to tape down the tubing)

It's also a good idea to stick with accessories and supplies sold by your pump's manufacturer and designed to work with your particular brand. Otherwise, it's like putting toner ink you bought on the street into your state-of-the-art laser printer. The results might not be very pretty.

You might wonder why we included needles and syringes in the list. They're there just in case. If something happens to the pump, you need to be able to give yourself insulin manually until you can fix the problem.

Puncturing the Pump Myths

One reason why pumps have been slow to catch on are all the myths surrounding them. Now's our chance to set the record straight.

Myth: The use of a pump requires a surgical procedure. Nope, just a quick five minutes to manually insert it.

Myth: The pump functions like an artificial pancreas. Not by a long shot. Pumps require regular care and maintenance and constant adjustments of the amount of insulin they're putting out to match up with your physical and emotional condition.

Myth: If I use a pump, I don't need to check my blood glucose levels as often. Wrong again. You still need to check your levels just as often as before to make sure your pump is working properly, hasn't clogged, and that you're managing insulin dosages properly. In fact, some insurance companies won't even approve a pump unless you can first show that you're pretty consistent at tracking your blood glucose levels.

Myth: If I'm using a pump, I don't have to worry about my diet. No way. You still to maintain a healthy diet that helps you maintain a healthy weight. You must learn how to count carbohydrates (to adjust the insulin dose), or, at the very least, eat a consistent amount of carbohydrates at each meal that matches up with the insulin dose you're taking.

Myth: With the pump, I will no longer experience any highs or lows of blood sugar. Sorry, no. Although you will probably have better overall control of your blood sugar after you get used to the pump, resulting in fewer episodes of hyperglycemia or hypoglycemia, you will still have a few. In fact, because there's no reservoir of insulin in your fat as there is with injections of long-acting insulin, if the pump stops working for some reason, the battery fails, you run out of insulin in the reservoir, or the catheter clogs or falls out, your blood sugar levels could get very high fairly quickly.

Myth: The pump makes it easier to lose weight and maintain a healthy weight. We wish it did, but the sad truth is that studies find that anything that better controls your blood sugar—whether frequent insulin injections or the pump—also results in weight gain unless you're really careful.

Myth: I'm less likely to get a skin infection with a pump than sticking myself with a needle all the time. Uh, no. At least a needle goes in and out quickly and, hopefully, is sterilized (along with the site to be stuck). But the cannula attached to a pump is inserted for a few days, increasing the possibility of infection or rashes (due to the tape) at the insertion site. That's why it's so important to change the site every two or three days.

Myth: I can throw away all my syringes, needles, and other insulin supplies. Ahh … better not. As we mentioned before, you also need to keep a stock of supplies on hand in case your pump malfunctions or, horrors, the battery dies.

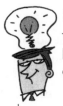

Sugar Sense _____

To prevent some of the disadvantages listed above, it's important to test your blood sugar levels at least four times a day if you have a pump. Here are other care tips:

♦ Change the catheter site every two to three days to minimize the risk of skin infections.

♦ If you have a rash at the catheter site, try creams containing aloe, vitamin E, or corticosteroids.

♦ Exercise and careful attention to what you eat can minimize the risk of weight gain.

So Why Bother?

So if there are so many disadvantages to the pump, why bother? Well, there are the medical reasons, discussed earlier. But there are many more reasons, as well.

For one, the pump can make it easier for you to exercise because it makes it easier to maintain good blood sugar levels during and after exercise. Studies in people with type 1 diabetes who use the pump find that it helps reduce the chances of low blood sugar that can arise after exercise, and it increases insulin sensitivity, both of which improve an individual's ability for aerobic exercise.

Plus, there are the emotional benefits. Some studies suggest that using a pump can result in less anxiety and depression over your diabetes, improve family dynamics, and provide a greater sense of control over your disease.

And let's not forget the flexibility. You don't have to worry about your blood sugar levels getting too high because your morning shot is wearing out and you haven't had a chance to run out for lunch and your lunchtime injection; instead, you can relax and get by on the basal drip until you get a chance to eat and get your bolus of insulin.

Say you want to unhook the pump while you go to your high-impact spinning class. You can unhook it, give yourself a dose of regular insulin, and head out for class.

Or say you're under a lot of stress at work, or your having your period (women often find their insulin needs increase when they're menstruating). Just slightly increase the amount of basal insulin you're receiving. When things even out, dial it back down again. Of course, you need to work out those dose changes with your doctor.

Living Life with a Pump

A pump sounds like a great idea until you start to grapple with the issues of daily life such as taking a shower or bath. Hey, it's not big deal. The pumps are designed to be easily disconnected from the tubing without having to remove the insertion end from your skin. Some manufacturers also have special bags that fit over the pumps so that you can keep them on while you bathe. Same thing goes for swimming. Many pumps today are safe for short periods of swimming.

If you're into more rugged sports such as snow boarding, mountain biking, or jet ski-ing, some manufacturers, such as Metronic's MiniMed, make hard protective cases that protect the pump from shock and water. And as long as the pump is kept under your clothes where it's warm, the insulin won't freeze.

Now about sex … don't worry. Pumps today come with long tubing so that they don't get in the way. And of course, you can always just "slip it off" as you "make yourself comfortable," and then plug it back in afterward during the cuddling part.

CAUTION **Warning**

Make sure that you don't expose your pump to high electromagnetic fields like those associated with MRI, x-rays, or CT scans. The high magnetic fields can affect the portion of the motor that regulates insulin delivery, causing too much insulin to be delivered. If you must have such a procedure, make sure to take off your pump and leave it outside the room. However, airline security devices are okay because the amount of radiation you're exposed to is delivered in such small doses.

Is a Pump Right for Me?

That's hard to say. As noted earlier, there's still some controversy over whether pumps are right for people with type 2 diabetes. Some experts recommend it only in the case of severe hypoglycemia and wide fluctuations in blood glucose levels. Others suggest that it might be as beneficial to those with type 2 as those with type 1. The answer really depends on your own individual circumstances, your medical team, your insurance, and so on. Check out the chart below to see if you might be a good candidate.

Is the Pump Right for Me?

Ideal Candidate for Pump if You ...	Probably Not Right for You if You ...
Are good at self-monitoring your blood glucose levels.	Can't stand to monitor your blood glucose levels.
Are capable of putting together and changing the infusion set.	Have mental or physical problems that would preclude you from maintaining the infusion set.
	Have a clear understanding of what's involved with diabetes self-care, including recognizing and tracking low blood sugars and infections.
Are very self-motivated to try it.	Are only trying it to please your family or healthcare team.
Have a skilled and enthusiastic healthcare team who wants to to see you try it.	Have a healthcare team that isn't supportive or fully trained in the use of pumps.

continues

Is the Pump Right for Me?   (continued)

Ideal Candidate for Pump if You ...	Probably Not Right for You if You ...
Are able to communicate effectively with your healthcare team.	Rarely admit when you're having health-related problems.
Have good health insurance to cover all or most of the costs.	Don't have good health insurance.
Can make simple calculations for carbohydrate counting.	Have problems reading or understanding what you read.
Don't mind other people knowing that you have diabetes.	Try to keep your condition hidden.

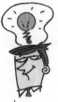

Sugar Sense

Wondering how to wear your pump? How about ...

- In your bra
- In small socks attacked to the inside of your clothes or underwear
- Clipped onto a garter belt
- Slipped into a pocket sewn on the inside of your bathing suit
- Slipped into the top of your pantyhose
- Sharing space with your cell phone in your belt holster (just keep the cell on top)
- In a little pocket sewn on your pillowcase (for those who like to sleep au natural)
- Pinned or clipped to your sheet
- In a fanny pack
- In your sock
- Under your hat (great for skiing or snowboarding!)

The Fine Art of Carbohydrate Counting

Using a pump requires that you remain aware of what you're eating, particularly those carbs. That's why most people using an insulin pump also have to use the carbohydrate-counting system described in Chapter 6. As a reminder, this requires that you figure out how many carbs each unit of insulin covers and bolus your pre-meal doses accordingly.

For instance, say you figure that one unit of insulin covers 15 grams of carbohydrates and lowers your blood sugar about 50 mg/dl. So if you're planning on a half bagel with a slice of cheese, and ¾ cup of blueberries for breakfast, that's about 30 grams of carbohydrates. Divided by 15, right there you need two units.

But you also have to take into account your existing blood sugar level. If your target level is 100, and it's 150 when you test before breakfast, then you need to add another unit. So your total dose would be three units.

These are the typical relationships for someone with type 1 diabetes who isn't over-weight and doesn't have much insulin resistance. If you have insulin resistance, how-ever, it has a large effect on these relationships. For instance, one unit of insulin will probably cover a smaller amount of carbohydrate and will lower your the blood sugar less. Just remember that every person is different, so you and your healthcare team have to determine which numbers are right for you.

And if you don't like math, stick with the injectable insulin! (Actually, some pumps today offer automatic carb calculators).

CAUTION

Warning

Don't press that button too soon. It's so easy to give yourself a bolus that you might be tempted to do it too soon before a meal. For instance, say you're eating out. Don't take the bolus before you get to the restaurant. What if you have to wait for a table or the kitchen is backed up? Better to settle in, order, and then give yourself a bolus. And of course, always make sure that you have some sugar with you in case hypoglycemia hits.

The Least You Need To Know

- ◆ Insulin pumps can provide flexibility and better blood sugar control in some patients.

- ◆ Insulin pumps are expensive and may not be covered by health insurance.

- ◆ Insulin pumps are not for everyone; you and your health care team need to think very carefully about whether you're a good candidate.

- ◆ Even with an insulin pump, you can still participate in sports activities and have a normal sex life.

Chapter 10

Alternative Approaches

In This Chapter

◆ All about complementary and alternative therapies

◆ Nutritional supplements

◆ Herbal supplements

◆ Hands-on therapies

This year, more than one in three Americans will use a natural or complementary healing method like acupuncture, herbal remedies, yoga, meditation, chiropractic, or massage, spending more than $21.2 billion—more than half out of their own pockets. Studies find that people with diabetes are twice as likely to use such therapies as people without—with nutritional and lifestyle advice, spiritual healing, herbal remedies, massage, and medication the most frequently used treatments.

But just because some television infomercial for an herbal product touting its "18 blood-sugar-lowering botanicals" catches your attention, that's no reason to reach for your pocketbook. Most of these therapies, particularly the supplements, are unproven; some can even harm you.

In this chapter, we focus on what you need to know about alternative remedies and how to find a reputable practitioner. We tell you what to stay away from, what might have some benefit, and what the existing research (what there is of it) shows. Although a big part of alternative therapies includes mind-body therapies like meditation and yoga, we save those for Chapter 12, when we talk about stress.

Welcome to the World of CAM

Why do Americans spend so much time and money on complementary or alternative therapies, also called CAM (Complimentary Alternative Medicine)? Experts who have scratched their head over this question and studied the issue point to numerous factors:

- **They're frustrated with conventional medications.** Face it, when even the most modern of medication still might not bring your blood sugar under control, it's tempting to look elsewhere.

- **They want something "natural."** Unfortunately, natural doesn't mean safe. We'll come back to this later.

- **They want a cure.** Dealing with a chronic disease like diabetes can be incredibly frustrating, and it's understandable that you might look outside traditional medicine for a cure. But it doesn't matter what kind of medicine you seek; with the exception of a pancreatic or islet cell transplant, there is no cure for diabetes, period.

- **They want to be in control.** This is a biggie. Today's healthcare system is often so large, so convoluted, and often so impersonal, that you can feel like a widget in a large widget factory rather than an individual who deserves personalized attention. Most CAM providers recognize this; they usually spend much more time with patients, and integrate the simple skill of listening into their treatment options.

- **They want to address what they perceive as the underlying cause of their illness.** Many alternative therapies are designed to reduce stress or "bolster a weak immune system." And there is some evidence showing that reducing stress can help control your diabetes (more about that in Chapter 12). So this is probably one of the best areas in which to seek CAM options if you have diabetes. However, as far as we know today, the immune system plays no direct role in type 2 diabetes.

♦ **They have cultural or spiritual beliefs.** Many other cultures have a long tradition of natural remedies and other alternative therapies; to them, our way of Western medicine is considered "alternative." This is particularly true of Eastern cultures.

Bet You Didn't Know

One of the few studies looking at the use of alternative remedies among those with diabetes found some interesting information:

♦ 57 percent of those with diabetes who used CAM discussed it with their regular physician.

♦ 43 percent of those who used CAM were actually referred to CAM providers by their physician.

♦ 21 percent of those with diabetes used spiritual healing, like seeing a clergy, praying, etc.), making it the second-most common form of CAM used.

What You Need to Know About CAM

Before we get into potential alternative treatments that may have some benefit for people with diabetes, you need to understand a few things about CAM:

♦ Never take anything, or undergo any therapy or treatment, without first letting your regular doctor know. Some herbal and nutritional supplements could interfere with medications you're taking, and some treatments might not be recommended if you have certain diabetes-related complications.

♦ Understand that there is far less scientific proof behind alternative remedies than behind traditional medications and procedures. The reasons for this lack of knowledge are many. Not only is it difficult to find funding to pay for well-designed studies on alternative remedies, it's often difficult to design such studies. Even the studies that have been conducted often have flaws. Plus, herbal products are rarely standardized; that is, there are different formulations with different strengths of active ingredients. Having said that, many alternative practices have thousands of years of use behind them; many have few, if any, side effects. Finally, there is something called "publication bias." Studies with negative findings are seldom published. That also is a likely reason why there is little published scientific proof for a beneficial effect of CAM in diabetes. CAM might not be very helpful in treating diabetes.

◆ Realize that the U.S. Food and Drug Administration (FDA) has a fairly hands-off approach to nutritional supplements and herbs. These products don't have to go through the rigorous testing and evaluation process required of over-the-counter and prescription drugs, and medical devices. The FDA doesn't even oversee their manufacturing to ensure purity as they do with pharmaceutical products. And even though the agency may receive reports of adverse events related to supplements and herbal products, it is very difficult for the FDA to have these products taken off the market.

Finding a Complementary or Alternative Provider

If you decide you want to try an alternative therapy, you should probably find a quality practitioner. In your search for a provider of alternative therapies, particularly herbal preparations, and other supplements, ask the following questions:

◆ What is the specific plan of treatment?

◆ What benefits can I expect and how long will it take?

◆ How will conventional medications be managed?

◆ How much will it cost?

◆ What are the possible side effects?

◆ Will you share information with my doctor?

Make sure your provider is licensed if your state requires it, or certified in his/her field by a respected professional organization. And make sure your regular physician knows who you're seeing and what you're doing. You may also be able to find an M.D. or a Doctor of Osteopathy (D.O.) who has received special training in complementary therapies. More physicians are learning more about these modalities so that they can better communicate with their patients.

Nutrition in a Pill

We covered the importance of a healthy diet in Chapter 6, but a few studies suggest that some nutritional supplements also may help maintain healthy blood sugar levels. Just remember that taking a vitamin or other nutritional supplement is no excuse for skimping on the nutrients you need to get the old-fashioned way, for instance, through food, nor does it enable you to change in any way the medications your doctor has prescribed.

One of the main uses of nutritional supplements is to reduce *oxidative stress*. What do we mean by this? Well, think about how apples turn brown once they're cut, and how a metal wagon left outside will rust. That's oxidative stress.

MedLingo

Oxidative stress refers to the damage caused to molecules in your body from **free radicals,** which are byproducts of normal chemical reactions.

Free Radicals and Other Nasty Things

Oxidative stress is the damage caused to the molecules of a substance, including our bodies, by nasty things called *free radicals*. Think of free radicals as the junk left over after the activities of normal living such as eating, breathing, and moving. They're like the pollution that results after you burn gasoline. Free radicals can also result from exposure to external sources, such as cigarette smoke, environmental pollutants, alcohol, radiation, and infections.

In your body, these free radicals tend to target blood fats like cholesterol, proteins, and DNA (the building blocks of genes), damaging the very structure of a cell and sometimes killing the cell. This in turn, damages tissues and organs. Today, oxidative stress is blamed in part for everything from dementia to heart disease.

Enter antioxidants. These "good guy" substances, primarily found in food sources, include the vitamins A, C, and E. In test tubes and animal studies, they have been found to protect cells from oxidative damage by destroying or modifying the free radicals, rendering them harmless.

Today researchers know that people with diabetes are prone to higher levels of oxidative stress. Some studies even suggest that low levels of dietary antioxidants may contribute to the development of type 2 diabetes. For sure, this oxidative stress affects heart health, because when LDL cholesterol particles become oxidized, they get smaller and denser, and are more likely to stick to coronary arteries, leading to heart disease. This may be one reason for the higher rates of heart disease in people with diabetes.

All that oxidative stress has led researchers to look at antioxidant supplements and foods that could help reduce oxidative stress as potentially helpful in people not only with diabetes but all of us, actually. However, so far there is not much evidence supporting their use.

Vitamin E

Studies testing vitamin E supplementation as a therapy to prevent various chronic diseases, including diabetes, have been disappointing. There have been six large clinical trials examining the affect of vitamin E on cardiovascular disease and/or diabetes control. None has shown a positive effect.

Most studies looked at vitamin E supplementation in combination with other nutrients. In one study, combining the amino acid L-arginine and the vitamins C and E improved blood vessel function in women with type 2 diabetes. The women took 1800 mg of vitamin E a day, a dose that no doctor would ever recommend, however. In fact, if you take vitamin E, you shouldn't take any more than 200 mg, or International Units (IU), a day.

Another study found that a combination of magnesium, zinc, vitamin C, and vitamin E taken daily for three months significantly decreased blood glucose levels in 69 people with type 2 diabetes. In this study, participants took the far safer dose of 150 mg of vitamin E. The same researchers did one other study and found that this combination also increased levels of "good" HDL cholesterol, low levels of which are a risk factor for heart disease. Of course, who knows whether it was the vitamin E or the other supplements that had the effect; researchers found no such reduction of glucose levels in people who only received vitamin E.

Besides the studies that did not show any effect, there is another reason to be cautious about taking high doses of vitamin E. One of the largest studies, which lasted the longest, found that vitamin E was associated with an increased chance of heart failure. Furthermore, when researchers combined all of the studies using vitamin E, not just those associated with diabetes, they found increased deaths in people taking doses of 400 or more IU per day.

Bottom line is this: if a multivitamin/mineral supplement is a regular part of your day to begin with, make sure yours does not contain more than 200 IU of vitamin E. On the other hand, if you don't want to take a vitamin pill, just make sure you're getting plenty of fruits and vegetables in your diet; they're chock full of vitamins and antioxidants.

Magnesium

Magnesium is a mineral that plays an important role not only in helping glucose get across cell membranes, but also in its metabolism within the cell. Low levels of magnesium are associated with an increased risk of insulin resistance and diabetes. One study conducted in 63 people with type 2 diabetes and low magnesium levels to start with found that supplementing with magnesium chloride resulted in lower fasting glucose levels and HgA1c levels than a control group who didn't receive supplements. Overall, however, studies looking at the impact on magnesium on blood sugar levels are mixed.

Bottom line is, supplementing with magnesium is generally safe. If you choose to supplement, about 400 mg a day should be sufficient. Much higher amounts could give you diarrhea. Good food sources of magnesium include dark-green leafy veggies, like spinach and kale, soy, legumes and seeds, nuts like almonds and cashews, whole grains and bananas, dried apricots, and avocados.

Warning

Don't supplement with magnesium if you have kidney disease. If your magnesium levels get too high (called *hypermagnesemia*), it could lead to a potentially fatal condition.

MedLingo

Hypermagnesemia is excess magnesium. Taking too much magnesium is particularly dangerous to people with kidney disease because they can't get rid of it normally and therefore it accumulates.

Chromium

Chromium is another important mineral. We need it for normal carbohydrate and fat metabolism. Chromium seems to work not only by increasing the number of insulin receptors on cells, but also by improving how they function.

Studies on the possible positive effects of chromium in people with diabetes are mixed, however. Some show an effect, while others don't. The inconsistency may be related to how much chromium is already in the body. Many people do not get enough chromium in their diet, especially older people. Furthermore, diabetes may cause the body to lose more chromium than if there were no diabetes. Thus, older people with diabetes are more likely to have a chromium deficiency. Unfortunately, it is not easy to measure the amount of chromium in the body, and so one can't be sure that there really is a chromium deficiency.

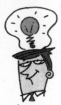

Sugar Sense _____

If you decide to try chromium, stick with chromium picolinate and chromium histidine. They are absorbed the best.

MedLingo _____

A **placebo** is a fake pill or treatment given to participants in clinical trials. It is made to look just like the real medication. Typically, neither patients nor doctors know whether patients are getting the real drug or a placebo in a clinical trial until the trial is over. This prevents bias from influencing the results.

In one large study involving 180 people with diabetes, one third received 200 mcg of chromium, one third received 1,000 mcg, and one third received a *placebo*. After four months, those receiving supplemental chromium had significantly lower HgA1C levels compared to those who didn't receive any. Those getting 1,000 mcg also had significant improvements in fasting blood glucose levels, two-hour glucose testing, and insulin and cholesterol levels. These were Chinese patients in whom a chromium deficiency may have been more likely. In general, positive studies have used at least 200 mcg of chromium a day. Studies using less have been mostly negative.

Bottom line is, chromium is considered a safe, potentially useful supplement for those with diabetes, but don't add it to your daily regimen without talking with your doctor first. You can also get good amounts of chromium in wheat germ, whole grains, brewer's yeast, and most meat. Generally, 200 to 400 mcg a day is plenty.

The Nutrient You Never Heard Of: Vanadium

Quick, raise your hand if you've ever heard of vanadium (or even know how to pronounce it.) Don't feel bad if your hand stayed by your side; vanadium is a little-known, nonessential trace nutrient that seems to play a role in the ability of cells to use glucose.

While a few small trials showed some benefits to vanadium use in people with type 2 diabetes (reduction in fasting blood sugar levels and HgA1C, and increased insulin sensitivity), they also showed some nasty side effects, including nausea, vomiting, gas, cramping, and diarrhea.

Bottom line is, skip the vanadium supplements.

L-carnitine

We talked a bit about L-carnitine earlier in this chapter as one of four supplements that, when taken together, seems to have some benefit for people with type 2 diabetes. L-carnitine is an amino acid that plays a role in fatty-acid oxidation. It's been the subject of numerous studies in recent years, leading some researchers to conclude that it may be a beneficial supplement for people with type 2 diabetes, both in terms of improving glucose use (because high levels of fatty acids in the blood interfere with glucose metabolism), and in preventing the diabetes-related heart condition known as *cardiac autonomic neuropathy.*

MedLingo

Cardiac autonomic neuropathy is a disease of the nerves that affects the heart.

Bottom line is, although there is no official recommendation on the use of L-carnitine in diabetes, studies find no side effects from its use. Talk to your doctor if you're interested in adding it to your daily regimen.

Alpha-Lipoic Acid

This potent antioxidant plays a role in carbohydrate metabolism and has been used to treat diabetic neuropathy for years in Germany. An overview of 15 studies on its use in people with diabetes found that the antioxidant improved glucose tolerance and reduced signs and symptoms of neuropathy.

Bottom line is, Alpha-lipoic acid appears to have some benefits for people with diabetes-related neuropathy. Talk to your doctor if you're interested in supplementing with it.

Bet You Didn't Know

Those chic edamame you've been popping at upscale restaurants are doing far more than providing a healthy pre-dinner snack; they're also benefiting your heart and possibly reducing insulin resistance. At least, that's what one study found, conducted on 32 women with type 2 diabetes. The women, all of whom controlled their diabetes with diet alone, added a supplement of phytoestrogens, (a plant-based estrogen found in soy) for 12 weeks. They also spent 12 weeks taking a placebo. When they were on the soy supplement, their insulin resistance, blood sugar control, and cholesterol levels improved enough to improve their overall risk of heart disease.

You can buy edamame fresh or frozen, and they're delicious with just a sprinkle of sea salt. Other good soy sources are soy burgers, tofu, soy crumbles, and soy milk (try it over cereal!).

Fish Oil

It seems the more we learn about fish oil the better it gets. Of course, our grandmothers knew that, which is why they always pushed cod liver oil, also known as fish oil, on our parents. Today, thankfully, we can get our fish oil in a manner that doesn't taste bad—just a couple of tasteless, easy-to-swallow gel capsules.

If you have diabetes, there's some evidence that supplementing with fish oil, a powerful antioxidant, could help prevent neuropathy, lower triglycerides and LDL cholesterol, and reduce your risk of heart disease.

Bottom line is, unless you're eating fish five times a week (and we don't actually recommend that because of high levels of mercury in many fatty fish), talk to your doctor about daily supplementation with fish oil.

A Hankering for Herbs

Before there were pills and shots, there were herbs. They were our first medicines, and many of our current remedies are derived from plants. Taxol, used to treat cancer? The Pacific yew tree. Aspirin? Originated from willow bark. Quinine, the first effective treatment for malaria? First found in the bark of another tree. So it should come as no surprise that various herbs may have some effect on diabetes control or complications.

But before you head for the herbal section of your health food store, we have a few caveats:

♦ The federal government does not regulate herbs, and doesn't guarantee their safety. There have been examples of dangerous contaminants turning up in herbal remedies, including lead found in one Indian remedy touted for people with diabetes. The contaminants often cause serious health problems or even death.

♦ Many herbal supplements contain little of the active ingredient on the label. If you want to try an herbal supplement, we recommend that you talk to your doctor and try to get the name of a trusted herbalist or naturopath who has been specially trained in the use of herbs and dispenses his or her own products.

♦ It's important to know the source of your supplement. Consumer Laboratories, Inc., independently tests supplements, providing information on hundreds of brands on its site, www.consumerlab.com. National Nutritional Foods

Association, an industry trade group, operates a *Good Manufacturing Practices (GMP)* certification program that includes inspections of manufacturing facilities to determine whether they meet specific performance standards, including staff training, cleanliness, equipment maintenance, record keeping, and receiving of raw materials. Once certified, manufacturers can then use NNFA's GMP seal on their products.

- Remember, supplements are still drugs. Just because they say "natural" on the label doesn't mean they're any safer than pharmaceutical drugs. It's still a chemical doing something in your body. So don't take higher-than-recommended doses, and don't take the supplement for longer than the recommended time period.

- Do your own research. To separate out the truth from the fiction, check out websites such as www.quackwatch.com, the American Council on Science and Health, www.acsh.org, and the National Council Against Health Fraud, www.ncahf.org.

- We can't say this too many times: Tell your doctor!

- Don't just take something just because your friend takes it; know *why* you're taking *what* you're taking.

MedLingo

Good Manufacturing Practices is a listing of regulations that describe the methods, equipment, facilities, and controls that are required for producing quality products. When you are purchasing products, look for products produced under these practices.

Warning

If you're breastfeeding or pregnant, skip the herbal remedies unless your doctor recommends them.

Herbal Remedies and Diabetes

Although literally hundreds of herbs have been used over the centuries to treat diabetes and diabetes complications, we focus on the few you tend to hear the most about. Keep in mind, however, that there are no studies directly comparing herbs against the drugs discussed in Chapters 7 and 8.

And studies find that the effects on your blood glucose from prescription medications are much greater than those found in the few positive studies evaluating the effect of herbs on diabetes. So don't change any medical therapy without first checking with your doctor.

♦ **American ginseng.** There are not a lot of studies, but one did suggest that this herb might reduce post-meal blood sugar spikes. If you do try it, take it with meals. Avoid it if you have high blood pressure, though; and don't take it near bedtime because it can cause insomnia.

MedLingo

Ayurvedic medicine is an ancient East Indian system of healing that seeks to promote balance through a healthy life-style and natural methods of healing

♦ **Fenugreek.** Fenugreek is actually a legume, belonging to the same family as peanuts! Its seeds are used to flavor foods, and it has been used as part of *Ayurvedic* medicine for centuries. Studies in humans and animals show that it may lower blood glucose, increase insulin sensitivity, reduce cholesterol levels, and increase HDL cholesterol. Don't take too much, though; it could give you gas!

♦ **Momortica Charantia,** also known as **bitter melon** or **balsam pear.** This plant is a climbing vine grown in Asia, Africa, and South and Central America. It's been used in folk medicine to treat diabetes for centuries. Various compounds have been isolated from its fruit, seeds, and seedlings and shown to have antidiabetic properties.

♦ **Gymnema sylvestra** is a woody, climbing vine found in central and southern India. Another traditional Ayurvedic remedy, Gymnema tastes sweet, resulting in its Hindi name, which means "destroyer of sugar." Water-based extracts of its leaves yield a series of acids that possess antidiabetic properties. In one study of 22 people with type 2 diabetes who were taking oral medications, supplementing with 400 mg/day of Gymnema for 12 to 18 months significantly reduced their blood glucose and HgA1C levels. Five of the patients were able to stop taking their oral medication altogether and just take the herb.

♦ **Pancreas Tonic.** This is a combination of 10 herbs that has been used in Ayurvedic medicine to treat diabetes. The herbs are aegle marmelose, pterocarpus marsupium, syzigium cumini, momordica charantia, gymnema sylvestre, trigonella foenum graecum, azadirachta, ficus racemose, tinospora cordfolia, and cinnamomum tamala. One study showed that this combination had a mild beneficial effect on people with type 2 diabetes who had very high blood sugars) but no effect on those in with only moderately high blood sugars.

◆ **Ginkgo biloba.** Ginkgo is an extract from one of the world's oldest trees, with individual trees living as long as 1,000 years. The extract comes from the leaves. It's an excellent antioxidant, and also protects nerve cells and improves blood vessel function. It's primarily used in diabetes for patients with *intermittent claudication*, or pain in the legs that comes on while walking as a result of *peripheral arterial disease*. The pain occurs during walking because that's when leg muscles need more oxygen, yet they can't get it because of clogged blood vessels in the legs. If this describes you, then talk to your doctor about adding it to your treatment regimen. One word of warning: Don't take it if you're on any kind of blood thinner, such as warfarin.

MedLingo

Intermittent claudication refers to the muscle cramps in the legs that occur with exercise and is one of the primary symptoms of **peripheral arterial disease** (PAD), also called **peripheral vascular disease** (PVD), a catch-all term for various problems caused by poor circulation due to clogged arteries in the legs.

On Pins and Needles: Acupuncture

You may know acupuncture as a therapy that involves someone sticking needles into you. That's just one very small part of it. The underlying principle behind acupuncture is that vital energy, or *Qi* (pronounced "chee"), flows along certain pathways in your body called *meridians*. When Qi is blocked, pain and illness result. Acupuncturists unblock *Qi* using hair-thin needles inserted at specific points in the body. They may, in some instances, use a laser beam that doesn't break the skin. They also might use very strong pressure with the hands instead of needles; this is called acupressure.

Each illness relates to certain acupuncture points that tend to be areas of decreased electrical resistance. This may be part of the scientific basis for acupuncture's effects. Also, studies find that acupuncture releases certain brain chemicals such as endogenous endorphins (think of runner's high) that reduce pain and discomfort.

That's why acupuncture appears to be an effective treatment for the pain of diabetic neuropathy, which, as you'll learn in Chapter 20, can be quite severe. In one study of 46 people with diabetes, most of whom were already taking standard medication for the pain, 6 acupuncture treatments over 10 weeks left most with significant improvement of their symptoms. And the effects seem to last; over the next three months to a year, 67 percent were able to stop using or reduce the amount of medicine they used to control the pain.

About 30 states have established training standards for certification to practice acupuncture, but not all states require acupuncturists obtain a license to practice. Although proper credentials don't necessarily translate to competency, they do indicate that the practitioner has met certain standards to treat patients with acupuncture.

The American Academy of Medical Acupuncture, www.medicalacupuncture.org, has a list of medical doctors who practice acupuncture. The National Acupuncture and Oriental Medicine Alliance, www.acuall.org, requires documentation of state license or national board certification from its listed acupuncturists. And the American Association of Oriental Medicine, www.aaom.org, can tell you the state licensing status of acupuncture practitioners across the United States as well.

> **Sugar Sense**
>
> Here's a good excuse to buy a hot tub. One study published in the prestigious New England Journal of Medicine looked at the effect of hot tubs on eight patients with diabetes who were asked to sit in the tub for 30 minutes a day for three weeks. During the study, the participant's weight, average blood glucose level, and average HgA1c levels decreased. Just make sure the water isn't too hot and that it's clean. Hey, check with your accountant; maybe you can deduct the spa as a medical expense!

Focusing With Biofeedback

Biofeedback is a therapeutic technique that teaches you how to control those unconscious physical responses, such as breathing, muscle tension, hand temperature, heart rate, and blood pressure. You achieve this control by learning to focus on and modify signals from your body. In diabetes, biofeedback has been primarily studied for its benefits in helping people with diabetes manage the pain of diabetic neuropathy.

These studies focus on a form of biofeedback called "thermal biofeedback," in which you are trained to increase the temperature of your legs by increasing blood flow to your legs. It sounds a bit weird, but studies conducted at the University of Virginia and other research centers find that people with diabetes, including those with mild to moderate autonomic and peripheral neuropathy, can deliberately increase their skin temperature using this process. This in turn, may improve blood pressure and blood flow in the legs resulting in pain-free walking in people with diabetes who also have intermittent claudication.

Studies find that you can generally learn this technique with one to four sessions of biofeedback; more sessions don't make a difference, so don't let your practitioner talk you into more. Biofeedback sessions generally cost between $50 and $80, and insurance may not cover the technique.

Although the practice isn't licensed, biofeedback therapists can receive certification from the Biofeedback Certification Institute of America (BCIA), at www.bcia.org, which also offers referrals to certified biofeedback therapists. BCIA estimates that about 2,000 healthcare professionals are certified either in general biofeedback, EEG biofeedback, or both.

Relaxing with a Massage

When you think massage, you may be thinking spa, expensive, indulgent. How about medical treatment? In fact, nearly three out of four people get massages to treat specific health problems for which they've already seen a doctor.

So what about for diabetes? We're pretty certain of one thing. A massage will definitely help you relax, and, as you'll read more about in Chapter 12, that alone can help improve blood glucose levels. It also can reduce blood pressure—and more than 70 percent of those with type 2 diabetes have high blood pressure.

However, there are few studies that show any benefit of massage on blood sugar management in people with type 2 diabetes. The couple that do exist, while they do show some benefit of massage on blood glucose control, aren't designed very well.

There is also some evidence, in people with type 1 diabetes, that massaging at the site of an insulin injection may result in a faster absorption of insulin. That in turn, could result in hypoglycemia.

So if you're planning a massage and you take insulin, make sure you tell the therapist that you have diabetes, and let him or her know about any signs of hypoglycemia. Also make sure you have something to eat or drink in case your blood sugar drops too low. And don't schedule a massage during the peak of insulin activity (see Chapter 9 if you need a reminder).

Twenty-nine states and the District of Columbia regulate massage therapists. Some local governments may also have some form of regulation. The primary national credential is the designation Nationally Certified in Therapeutic Massage and Bodywork, or NCTMB. To find a therapist in your area, click on the American Massage Therapy Association's website locator: www.amtamassage.org/findamassage/locator.htm.

The Least You Need to Know

◆ People with diabetes are twice as likely as those without the disease to use complementary and alternative therapies.

◆ The U.S. Food and Drug Administration has very little oversight over the production and sale of nutritional and herbal supplements.

◆ A few nutritional and herbal supplements may have some benefit for people with diabetes.

◆ Therapies like massage, acupuncture, and biofeedback may have some benefits for people with diabetes, but the studies showing this are few and poorly designed.

◆ Always tell your doctor about any CAM therapies you're trying.

Part 3

Daily Living with Diabetes

In this section, you learn about the nitty-gritty, day-in-and-day-out issues of living with diabetes. That means monitoring your blood glucose levels in Chapter 11, getting enough sleep and managing stress and any illnesses in Chapter 12, and understanding any changes that may or may not occur in your sex life. We also tell women considering pregnancy what they can expect, and give you some pointers for managing your career when you have diabetes.

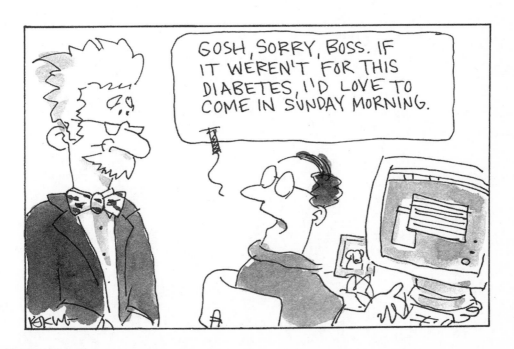

Chapter 11

Monitoring Your Levels

In This Chapter

◆ Choosing a glucose meter

◆ Ensuring accuracy

◆ When and how to test

◆ Other diabetes tests

As discussed previously, one of the keys to effectively managing diabetes is regular self-testing of your blood glucose, also known as SMBG, or *self-monitoring of blood glucose*.

There are many kinds of tests that track your blood glucose levels, but this is the only one that will give you real-time information on a daily basis, enabling you to modify your diet, medications, and exercise regimen accordingly. In this chapter, we'll tell you how to choose and use a glucose monitor, and, most important, how to incorporate it into your life so you can better manage your diabetes.

Before There Were Meters

Prior to the first meters, the only home test available to people with diabetes was the urine test. You either dip chemical test strips or place tablets into, well, your pee, to check for high blood sugar. These urine tests have a lot of problems:

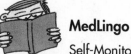

MedLingo

Self-Monitoring of Blood Glucose (SMBG) refers to home testing of your glucose levels using a glucose meter.

MedLingo

Ketones are chemicals that your body produces when it breaks down fat for energy because there isn't enough insulin in your blood.

- For the tablet test, accurate mixing is critical; you have to use precise amounts of urine and water.

- They sometimes fail to detect high levels of blood sugar, particularly in older people and in anyone with kidney damage or high levels of *ketones* in their urine.

- They don't give you your blood sugar level at the time of the test, only an approximate level over the past few hours when the urine collected in your bladder, in other words, from the last time you emptied your bladder until the time you took the sample for the urine test.

- They can't tell you if your blood sugar is low, because at lower levels, glucose doesn't enter your urine.

- Glucose levels change depending on the volume of urine; for instance, if you're a big water drinker, the volume of water can be a problem in accurately determining the amount of glucose.

Today, urine tests are used only by people who, for whatever reason, are unable to use a home glucose meter.

Just a Bit of History

Although the first glucose meter was patented in 1971, the first meter didn't hit the market until a decade later. They were large, expensive, and challenging to use.

Pretty quickly, however, doctors realized that home blood glucose meters could revolutionize diabetes management. For the first time, it put blood sugar control right in the hands of the patient, both an empowering and a frightening thing to do.

Still, it took until 1986 before the American Diabetes Association, the Centers for Disease Control and Prevention, the Food and Drug Administration, and the National Institutes of Health, all the big guns in health policy, got together at a conference and recommended that patients use SMBG.

It Works, It Really Works!

The next major event in the world of SMBG for those with type 2 diabetes was the publication of the Kumomoto study in 1995. This small Japanese study clearly showed for the first time that tight control of blood glucose, made possible with home meters, could significantly reduce the risk of diabetes complications in people with type 2 diabetes who used insulin. A much larger study published in 1998, called the United Kingdom Prospective Diabetes Study (UKPDS), confirmed these results.

During the UKPDS study, people with type 2 diabetes who maintained tight control of their blood glucose levels reduced their HbA1c levels and their risk of small blood vessel complications by 25 percent. Many of them, especially those requiring insulin, used SMBG.

The jury is still out on the benefits of SMBG in those who control their diabetes with oral medications or diet and exercise. Potentially, knowing your blood sugars can help educate you about how different foods affect you, if you test after eating. If you find your levels are high, it might motivate you to follow your diet better and exercise more.

However you do it, there is no doubt whatsoever that the better you control your blood sugar, the better you're going to feel in the long run and the less chance you have of getting the small blood vessel complications, like eye, kidney, and peripheral nerve diseases, so common in those with diabetes.

Join the (Still-Small) Crowd

These days, having diabetes and not owning at least one glucose meter makes you as out of step with the times as an audiophile who still listens only to vinyl records. Owning two or three is even better, because then you can always have one nearby, wherever you go.

Owning a meter is just the first step, however. You still have to test. And unfortunately, national data shows that barely one fourth of those with type 2 diabetes tested their blood at least once a day.

In fact, a study published in 2001 looking at data from 1988 to 1994 found that 29 percent of patients treated with insulin, 65 percent of those treated with oral medications, and 80 percent of those treated with diet alone had never monitored their blood glucose, or monitored it less than once a month. Only a third of those taking insulin and 5 to 6 percent of those taking oral mediations or treating their condition with diet alone monitored it daily.

So why don't more people test their blood sugar?

Well, it's expensive, for one thing. Meter costs range from a low of $10 up to $200 or more, and each test strip can cost as much as 50 cents each. That adds up if you're testing three or four times a day. Although Medicare and most health insurances cover the costs, if you don't have health insurance, or you don't have a policy that covers meters and testing supplies, you're in trouble.

> **Sugar Sense**
>
> Your health insurance plan should cover the cost of a new meter every year. Plus, most meter manufacturers offer huge rebates, often giving you the meter for nearly free. The reason? Just like printer manufacturers, they make their money on the supplies, not the machine itself. So look around for the best deal on the meter you want. And ask your doctor to loan you one to test before committing. Most endocrinologists have sample meters for you to try in their offices.
>
> If you don't have insurance, check out eBay for some great deals on meters and supplies.

Another reason that more people with diabetes don't use meters is that neither they nor their healthcare providers get enough education about the importance of testing, its health benefits, or how to use the results. For the providers, it's also often a matter of time. It takes time to analyze the results and train patients. But if you're going to the trouble of testing, you should know how you're doing. So ask your doctor nicely, but firmly, to provide feedback on the results.

Then there's that needle thing; sticking yourself several times a day, especially if you're already taking insulin, definitely isn't anyone's idea of a fun time. Plus, speaking of time, people with diabetes sometimes think that it's just going to take too much time to do this kind of testing.

That's a shame. Because these days, there's no easier way to monitor your blood glucose levels. It doesn't have to hurt, and there are ways to handle the cost.

Your first step is picking the right meter.

Meters, Meters; Who's Got the Meters?

Today, there are more than 30 glucose meters on the market and it seems that the features and styles change as often as those in automobiles.

Today's meters do everything short of sorting, washing, and folding your laundry. They can take your blood sugar without pricking your skin; beep to remind you when it's time to test; automatically beam the results to your computer (and then send them to your doctor's computer). They can be used with the traditional fingerstick, or you can take samples from other, less-painful parts of your body.

Some are one-step meters, requiring just one step to take the blood, test it, and display the results. Some can be used one-handed; others provide blood ketone testing as well as glucose testing, use sensor cartridges instead of individual test strips, and give you results in as little as three seconds.

Some can be used outside when it's as cold as 32 degrees or as hot as 122 degrees; others require more temperate temperatures to work.

There are certain basics you need to consider when you're choosing a meter, however:

- Amount of blood needed for each test. Obviously, the less the better because less blood means easier finger sticks. Some meters can now test with a drop of blood as miniscule as the period at the end of this sentence.

- Testing speed. How long does it take to get a reading?

- Size. Some are the size of a pager, others the size of a wallet or larger. Also take into consideration your eyesight: Can you clearly read the digital readout? If not, some meters even provide audio instructions and results.

- Ability to store test results in memory. This is critical. You don't want to be rushing off to your computer or scribbling on little slips of paper every time you test. It's still important, though, to keep a paper record in a log book you should get from your doctor's office. The memory feature enables you to download the results to your computer or even your doctor's computer, or, in some instances, to print them out.

- Cost. As we mentioned before, this varies considerably.

- Cost of the test strips or cartridges.

◆ Measurement range. Most glucose meters are able to read glucose levels over a broad range of values from as low as 0 to as high as 600 mg/dL. The range differs among meters, however, so be careful as to how you interpret very high or low values. In other words, if you get an extremely high or low reading from your meter, confirm it with another reading and consider checking your meter's calibration.

Testing Without Needles

How cool is this? Today you can wear a watch-like device on your wrist that tests your blood sugar levels without needles. Called the GlucoWatch G2 Biographer, it consists of two parts: the "watch" part and the "auto sensor." The watch is worn on your arm and displays and stores the results from the test performed by the auto-sensor.

This device, manufactured by Cygnus, Inc., uses a process called *reverse iontophoresis*. The GlucoWatch can be programmed to automatically test your glucose levels every 10 minutes, beeping at you if your levels are too high or too low.

You still have to calibrate the GlucoWatch device using a fingerstick, and it is designed to be used as an adjunct to regular glucose meters, not as a stand-alone product. It has to "warm up" for several hours before you can use it and the reading isn't "real time," but rather, provides a sense of what your glucose *was* 10 to 20 minutes earlier.

Other downsides? Reports of skin irritation, itching, redness, and blistering. Plus, if you sweat a lot, it may throw off your reading. And it's not cheap; the GlucoWatch Biographer costs about $800, with the sensor costing about $9 each. The device itself does require a prescription.

Another needleless device, also requiring a prescription, is the Lasette Laser Lancing device, which uses a laser beam to vaporize the tissue to collect the blood sample. This one costs even more than the GlucoWatch, about $1,500 for the device and $60 for two cartridges, 120 uses per cartridge. Unfortunately, it still hurts!

MedLingo

Reverse iontophoresis is a process in which a low electric current is used to move glucose through your skin for testing in a special meter.

Bet You Didn't Know

Whoever thought the tip of the finger was the ideal place to get blood must not have known that you have more nerve endings in the tip of your fingers than in nearly any other part of your body. Ouch!

A third device, called the MiniMed CGMS System Gold, consists of a tiny tube, or catheter, inserted just under the skin. The catheter collects a small amount of liquid that is passed through a "biosensor" that measures the amount of glucose present.

This device, also available by prescription only, is not intended for regular glucose monitoring, just for occasional use to discover trends in sugar control.

> ### Bet You Didn't Know
>
> Eventually, glucose testing with lancets may become a thing of the past. Researchers are investigating numerous other methods, including shining a beam of light onto your skin, measuring the energy waves your body emits, applying radio waves to your fingertips, using ultrasound, or checking the thickness of fluids under your skin.

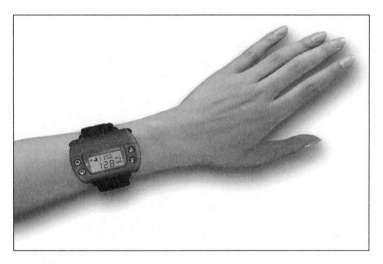

The GlucoWatch G2 Biographer meter. ©Cygnus, Inc.

Where Do You Want to Test Today?

In the old days, about five years ago, you only had one choice when it came to glucose testing: finger sticks. Some people, particularly those with type 1 diabetes who had to test numerous times a day, pricked their fingers so often they got calluses and lost the feeling in their fingertips.

Luckily, glucose meter manufacturers caught on, and today there are "alternative site testing" models that enable you to sample blood from other locations, including the upper arm, forearm, base of the thumb, abdomen, and thigh, which are generally less painful.

This sounds great, but it comes with some caveats. The primary one is that blood tested in other parts of your body may show different levels of glucose. How can this be? Well, it seems there's a reason why finger sticks were the original site selected way back when. Blood in the fingertips show changes in glucose levels more quickly than blood in other parts of the body.

That's why the FDA requires that manufacturers of alternative site meters warn you to use samples from your fingertip if …

◆ You think your blood sugar is low.

◆ You are not aware of symptoms when you become hypoglycemic.

◆ The site results do not agree with the way you feel.

Bet You Didn't Know

Have a problem with a meter? Almost all companies have customer-service staff available 24 hours a day for you to call in case of a problem. You can also report problems with glucose meters and other medical devices to the FDA through its MedWatch program. Just go to the following link online, www.fda.gov/medwatch/how.htm, for instructions on reporting problems. Keep in mind, however, that the FDA is not going to be able to help you with your problem; they're just collecting information.

Sugar Sense

It's important to wash your hands before testing. Any kind of sugary residue on your hands could throw your results off. Also, make sure you dry them well; otherwise the blood won't form into a good drop but will spread out across the tip of your finger, making it difficult to get it onto the strip.

Getting It Right

Meters are only as good as the information you receive from them. If they're not calibrated properly, or if you're not using them properly, then the levels you measure won't be accurate.

In one study of 280 patients with type 1 and type 2 diabetes, for instance, about one in five had meters that weren't accurate. Among the most common reasons for the problem were lack of periodic meter evaluation, incorrect use of control solutions to calibrate the meter, lack of hand washing, and unclean meters.

That's why it's so important to calibrate your meter. With some meters, this can be done automatically; others require that you use special chips, strips, or solutions.

You should also take your meter into your doctor's office at least once a year to ensure that the results you get match the results in a quality laboratory.

Sugar Sense

If you switch brands of glucose meters, make sure you overlap their use. In other words, use both for a few days and compare the results, because one may give you a higher reading than the other.

When to Test

You need to talk to your doctor and other members of your health-care team to determine the right testing schedule for you. If you're taking insulin, your doctor will likely ask you to test before meals and your bedtime snack. Without this information, doctors can't adjust your insulin doses very well.

If you're not taking insulin, testing before and one to two hours after a meal can be helpful. The difference between the two values tells you how the food you ate affected your blood sugar. This will provide you with a good sense of what you should eat, or, put another way, what you *shouldn't* eat. Of course, keep in mind that it's often the amount, or portion size, of what you're eating that's to blame for blood sugar spikes.

Bet You Didn't Know

It's always a good idea to have a small snack before you go to sleep if you're taking insulin in order to avoid overnight hypoglycemia.

Testing before and after you exercise can tell you how this important activity affects your blood sugar, helping you and your doctor determine the type and amount of exercise best for you.

There are other times you'll want to test more often, however:

Sugar Sense

Avoid anything that keeps you from testing. For instance, if you live in a two-story house, get a second meter to keep upstairs. Keep an extra meter at your office and even one in your car. But if you're using more than one meter, stick to one brand so the results are consistent.

- When you're sick. As you'll learn in Chapter 12, when you're sick your blood glucose levels often run high.

- If your diabetes medication changes or you add other medications.

- If you switch insulin regimens.

- If you change your diet.

- If you change your exercise or physical activity regimen. For instance, if you take a vacation that involves more physical activity than you're used to.

- If the stress in your life increases (e.g., if you're going through a divorce).

- If you have symptoms of hypoglycemia or hyperglycemia.

How to Test

So now that you've picked out your meter, brought it home, and taken it out of the box, what's next? Read the instructions! Every meter has different instructions for testing. Most manufacturers also provide toll-free numbers and in-depth websites for information (see Resources). Many doctors have nurses in their offices who can show you how to use the meter.

There are some general instructions for testing regardless of the meter that you use, however:

1. Wash your hands with soap and warm water, not cold; the warm water helps bring blood to the surface. Dry completely. Or, if you're not near a water source, clean the area with alcohol and dry completely. Make sure that the alcohol is entirely gone; otherwise it will sting if any gets under your skin. You also can use one of those alcohol-based, antibacterial hand cleaners.

MedLingo

A **lancet** is a small device with a sharp needle on the end used to prick the skin for blood tests.

2. Prick your fingertip using a *lancet*. These are usually put into a spring-loaded device so all you have to do is place the platform on your fingertip and push a button.

3. After the lancet pricks your finger, hold your hand down and squeeze your finger until a small drop of blood appears. Put the drop of blood on the test strip. For some meters, the strip will already be in the machine; for others, the strip should be inserted only after you've placed the drop on it.

4. Follow the instructions for inserting the test strip and using the meter.

5. Record the test result in your log book.

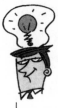

Sugar Sense

If you have delicate skin, choose a lancet with a longer cover (which means a shorter needle) for shallower penetration. You also can find lancet devices that offer several different settings for penetration, from shallow to deep. This is important because you may find you need different penetrations depending on the site for testing and the temperature of your skin.

Best bet are automatic lancing devices that use a spring-loaded action to pierce the skin.

Aiming for the Right Level

So now that you've got this testing thing down, what's your goal? What should your blood sugar be? Finally, we have a pretty specific answer for you.

Based on the UKPDS we mentioned earlier, the American Diabetes Association recommends that most adults with type 2 diabetes aim for glucose levels between 90-130 mg/dl *before* meals and below 180 mg/dl *after* meals.

Now, as they say in e-mails, YMMV (your mileage may vary). If you're subject to severe hypoglycemia, are elderly, or get sick often, then those levels may need to be adjusted. That's why it's so important to stay in regular contact with your doctor.

Tracking the Results

Today, tracking the results of your blood testing is easier than ever. Most meters have computer memories that can store dozens, even hundreds of test results. Several enable you to download them to your computer and upload them to online programs that can provide nifty charts and graphs putting all those numbers into perspective.

Still, just to be on the safe side, you should still maintain a log book. This is a book, usually available from your healthcare provider, that provides room to write your results and your activities (eating, sleeping, exercising, etc.) around that test. After all, meters get lost, destroyed, break, and so on, and you don't want three weeks of results to be wiped out into nothingness.

More important, your comments will enable your doctor to judge whether certain values should be considered in his or her treatment decisions. For instance, suppose you are taking a sulfonylurea or insulin and have a low glucose value, but your comments show that you missed a meal. Without that comment, your doctor might think that you're taking too much medication, resulting in the low glucose levels.

The Care and Feeding of Your Glucose Meter

You wouldn't buy a new cell phone and then just toss it in the garbage heap, would you? Well, your glucose meter deserves the same love and attention you'd heap on any new electronic device. That means regular cleaning, usually with soap and water, using only a dampened cloth over the sensitive parts.

You also need to be aware of factors that may affect your glucose meter and how well it functions. This, in turn, could affect the accuracy of your results. These include the following:

- ◆ Vitamin C. In some meters, high blood levels can result in falsely high readings.

- ◆ Altitude. Higher altitude results in less oxygen in your blood, which could lead to falsely low results.

- ◆ Temperature. Some meters won't function properly if it's too hot or too cold.

- ◆ Humidity. Even the humidity in the bathroom could affect the performance of the test strips, as can wet hands.

- ◆ Test strips. Only use the strips recommended for your particular meter, and make sure they haven't expired. It is also important to keep the vial containing the strips closed so that they don't get wet or dry, which could affect accuracy.

Testing at Your Doctor's Office

So if you're doing all this testing at home, why does your doctor still need to test you in the office? To be on the safe side. Face it, the testing equipment in your doctor's office is far more precise than the little glucose meter you carry around in your purse or suit jacket. Think of it as insurance that your own meter is working properly.

Plus, your doctor is going to do some tests that you can't easily do at home. These tests will provide more information than just the level of your blood sugar at that point in time.

And, if your doctor is doing the test, he or she knows that the results will be accurate, tried and true. No cheating!

No Place to Hide: Glycated Hemoglobin Testing

If you think you can fool your doctor into thinking you've been good with one or two individual blood glucose meters, think again. These days, your doctor has the glycated hemoglobin test. It goes by a bunch of monikers, including glycosylated hemoglobin, glycohemoglobin, HbA1c, or A1C. For simplicity's sake, we're going to keep calling it the HbA1c, as we've done throughout the book.

The HbA1c works like a kind of time traveler, providing you and your doctor with a picture of your glucose levels over the past three months or so.

The test measures the amount of glucose attached to *hemoglobin* molecules. Over time, some of the glucose in your blood binds, or attaches, to hemoglobin. Once it's bound, it's called the hemoglobin A1c, and the amount is directly related to your average level of blood glucose for the past three to four months.

The American Diabetes Association recommends the test four times a year if you use insulin, and at least twice a year if you don't. Your healthcare team may have its own preferences.

Sugar Sense

Make sure you bring your blood glucose meter with you to the doctor's office. Then you can do your own test on your blood sugar when the technician tests yours. Making sure the two match up lets you know that your meter is working properly.

MedLingo

Hemoglobin is the part of red blood cells that carry oxygen.

Someone without diabetes would have a level between 4 and 6 percent; so, the closer you are to 6 percent, the better you're doing. The chart below shows how your HbA1c compares to the average daily blood glucose level.

Here's how your HbA1c compares to the average blood glucose level over the past three months:

Comparing Apples and Oranges

HbA1c (%)	Average blood glucose (mg/dl)
6	135
7	170
8	205

continues

Comparing Apples and Oranges (continued)

HbA1c (%)	Average blood glucose (mg/dl)
9	240
10	275
11	310
12	345

As you can see, every 1 percent change in your HbA1c level reflects a 35 mg/dl change in your average blood glucose level.

Bet You Didn't Know

If you have an iron deficiency anemia (caused by heavy bleeding from your period or bleeding from another part of your body), sickle cell anemia, or other conditions that affect how long your red blood cells hang around in your bloodstream, you may wind up with a falsely low HbA1c reading. Make sure you doctor knows about any of these blood-related conditions.

There are a couple of FDA-approved home HbA1c tests. They generally require that you put a drop of blood (you get that the same way you do for SMBG) on a strip, and then send it to the manufacturer. Your results are either posted online, mailed, phoned, or faxed to you and/or your doctor. With the most recent FDA-approved HbA1c test, you can do the test yourself at home. But since you only need to get the test done every three months or so, this may not be a wise investment because your health insurance should cover it in your doctor's office.

MedLingo

Glycosylated means the binding of glucose to protein products. **Albumin** is a protein produced by the liver and found in plasma, the liquid part of the blood.

Fructosamine Test

If the HbA1c is a long-term look at your blood sugar, and the home glucose monitor is a real-time look, then the fructosamine test is a mid-range glimpse, providing information about the past two to four weeks. The test measures the amount glucose linked to proteins, primarily *albumin*, in your blood, which forms *glycosylated* products.

High values mean that your blood glucose was high over the past couple of weeks. This test is best for monitoring short-term changes in your blood sugar levels during pregnancy, or after major changes in your treatment plan.

If you're scheduled for this test, stay away from vitamin C supplements for a day. High levels can interfere with accurate readings.

Ketone Tests

As we discussed earlier, if your body doesn't have enough insulin, and thus can't get glucose into cells for energy, it begins burning fat for energy. This, in turn, releases acids called ketones, which are poisonous to body tissue.

Ketones pass through your body in your urine, which is why a urine test is often used to test for them. High levels of ketones can result in diabetic ketoacidosis, which we talked about earlier, leading to nausea, vomiting, abdominal pain, and, potentially, coma and death.

With type 2 diabetes, you usually don't have to test for ketones unless you're sick, under a lot of stress, or have ketoacidosis-like symptoms.

You can test with a urine test using dipsticks or a home blood test. For now, each is considered equally reliable. However, since a build-up of ketones in people with type 2 diabetes happens so rarely, most doctors won't ask you to test for them.

Identifying Kidney Disease Early: Microalbumin Test

Another test your doctor should perform is for low levels of albumin in your urine. This protein only appears in your urine if your kidneys aren't working well. If a small amount is found in the urine, you have *microalbuminuria*. It's important to know your levels because there is a medication available that can prevent your kidneys from getting worse. It may even return them to normal! We'll talk more about this in Chapter 18.

There are a few home albumin-testing kits on the market today, in which you take a urine sample and mail the test to a laboratory, which provides the results. Always share the results of any home test with your doctor.

MedLingo

Microalbumin is a protein that, if released into the urine, may indicate early kidney disease.

The Least You Need to Know

- ◆ Buy a glucose meter that works best for your lifestyle.

- ◆ Calibrate your glucose meter as often as the directions recommend.

- ◆ Test as often as your doctor recommends.

- ◆ Make sure that you also get tested in your doctor's office, particularly for your HbA1c levels.

The Three S's: Stress, Sleep, and Sickness

In This Chapter

- ◆ All about stress
- ◆ Stress and your blood sugar levels
- ◆ Managing stress
- ◆ A good night's sleep
- ◆ When you're sick

Stressed much? If you're like most Americans, you spend most of your life in a constant state of hyperalertness, multitasking like there's no tomorrow, rushing from one item on your to-do list to another, and coping with a continual barrage of frustrations, annoyances, and problems. These all contribute to a stress level nearly certain to affect your health—and your blood sugar levels.

Stress: The Good, the Bad, and the Ugly

Defining stress is, well, downright stressful. First of all, it's important to understand that not all stress is bad. Good things happening in your life such as a job promotion, a marriage, or the birth of a much-wanted child are all stressful events.

Basically, stress is any event—internal or external to your body—that results in the release of certain hormones called stress hormones. These include *epinephrine* (also called *adrenaline*), *norepinephrine* (also called *noradrenaline*), and *cortisol*. Not only can stress significantly affect your ability to control your blood sugar, as you'll see in a minute, but it also significantly increases your risk for some of the already-increased risks associated with diabetes, namely heart disease, high blood pressure, and depression.

MedLingo

Epinephrine (adrenaline), norepinephrine (noradrenaline), and **cortisol** are hormones released when you are under stress.

Hans Selye, M.D., the Austro-Hungarian-born Canadian physician and physiologist, was the first modern researcher to describe the effects of stress on our health, and even he spent much of his life trying to come up with an adequate definition for the word "stress." The best he could do was, "the rate of wear and tear on the body."

Since then, researchers have made a bit of progress on the linguistic front, defining three primary forms of stress:

- **Acute stress.** This is the most common form of both good and bad stress. A marriage proposal, the birth of a baby, and a promotion at work are all forms of "good" acute stress. A car accident, a robbery, even a traffic ticket represent the "bad" forms of acute stress.

- **Acute episodic stress.** Although acute stress is generally situational, acute episodic stress comes when these situations continue unabated. Someone who is chronically late, lives from one deadline to another, and is constantly overwhelmed is living with acute episodic stress.

- **Chronic stress.** There is no such thing as "good" chronic stress. This kind of stress is the stress of poverty, dysfunctional families, or being trapped in an unhappy marriage or a despised job or career. It's a grinding, day-in-and-day-out stress that eventually wears you down.

The latter two types of stress—acute episodic and chronic—are responsible for much of the physical and emotional damage caused by stress. In fact, the American Psychological Association reports that 43 percent of adults suffer adverse health effects from stress, and 75 to 90 percent of all physician office visits have stress-related components.

Your Body on Stress

So why does getting frustrated at a traffic jam, racing to meet a deadline, or going through a divorce have physical repercussions? Blame the way we're hard-wired.

To understand the connection between stress and blood glucose levels, you need to return to our ancestral beginnings, to the biological underpinnings that made us what we are today.

Back then, we needed stress to give our bodies the extra "oomph" it needed to get the heck out of the way of that two-ton mammoth or charging lion. So we evolved so that any time the brain senses that the body is in danger, it jumps into action, releasing hormones that trigger a cascade of effects on your body that enable you to run like the wind or give you the wherewithal to stay and fight.

The first step in the process (whether the initial cause is as mild as a traffic jam or as horrific as a diagnosis of cancer) is the release of those stress hormones. Hormones, you might remember, deliver messages to other parts of the body and these are no exception. They tell your liver to release stored sugar and your fat cells to release fatty acids to give your muscles a quick burst of energy for that fight-or-flight reaction.

At the same time, they signal your lungs to expand to take in more oxygen, your heart to beat faster, and your blood pressure to rise so that more oxygen-rich blood heads throughout your body. Other signals go out to your bowel and intestinal muscles so they contract, which causes blood to leave your abdominal area and head to where it can really do some good (that's one reason stress might leave you feeling nauseous and often has such a major impact on your digestive system).

The result is stress-related conditions ranging from chronic hypertension, chest pain, and heartburn to constipation and irritable bowel syndrome, depression, anxiety, and fatigue. It can also make you fat. Cortisol is not only a powerful appetite trigger, but chronically high levels of cortisol actually stimulate the fat cells inside your abdomen to fill with more fat, creating a life-threatening form of fat called *visceral fat*, which is associated with insulin resistance and puts you at higher risk for heart disease and diabetes. Not only that, but cortisol also causes the liver to produce more glucose (although not as quickly as the other stress hormones).

MedLingo

Visceral fat is located around the organs inside the belly and, as such, is deeper in the body than subcutaneous fat, which lies under the skin. Increased levels of visceral fat have been associated with insulin resistance, the metabolic syndrome (discussed later in the chapter), and cardiovascular disease.

All of which can play havoc with your blood sugar levels, especially if you have diabetes.

Diabetes and Stress: The Connection

So, okay, you've encountered a stressor (you've just been told you're losing your job). This is no raging, out-of-control lion, but that doesn't matter. Your body still reacts in the same way because this incident is perceived as a threat.

So now you have all this extra glucose in your blood (which came from your liver) prepared to feed energy to your muscles. If you didn't have diabetes, that wouldn't be much of a problem; the signals in your body are working properly and your pancreas gets the message that it needs to kick up insulin production a notch to get that glucose into muscle cells. But you *do* have diabetes; thus, things *aren't* working properly.

So all this blood sugar is wandering around your bloodstream, knocking on muscle cells but getting nowhere. Plus, the more stress you're under (not only are you losing your job, but your wife is leaving you, your son just failed geometry, and your car is on its last legs), the higher your levels rise.

Stress can affect your diabetes control in other ways, too. For instance, what's the first thing most people turn to when they're stressed? Alcohol, cigarettes, and food, right? And the food? It's often high-sugar, high-fat comfort foods. (Anyone for a gallon of double-chocolate Haagen Daz or a serving of cheese fries?)

Also if you're stressed, you might not feel like exercising or tracking your blood sugar levels closely. Plus, studies find that chronic stress increases your risk of de-pression, which is already fairly prevalent in people with diabetes.

Tackling the Stress

So what should you do? After all, there's no way to get rid of all the stress in your life (and if you did, it would be a pretty boring life). Plus, even "good" stress, such as a job promotion, can have similar effects on your body.

Face it, stress in your life is here to stay.

What you can change, however, is how you *react* to the stress in your life. A growing body of evidence finds that people with diabetes who learn and use stress management techniques such as progressive muscle relaxation, biofeedback, mental imagery, deep breathing, and other techniques can significantly improve their blood sugar levels over the long term.

In fact, one major study published in the journal *Diabetes Care* in January 2002 found that these simple stress-management techniques can lower blood sugar levels in people with diabetes enough to reduce their risk for many diabetes-related complications.

It might not work for everyone—follow-up studies show mixed results, particularly in highly anxious people with diabetes—but it's certainly worth a try.

Sugar Sense

What kind of personality do you have? Are you the kind of person who goes out of your way to do for others, ignoring your own needs in the process? Or one who focuses on yourself first, and then the rest of the world? Well, even though it might sound counterintuitive, it turns out that your blood sugar level might be better off if you put yourself first more often. One study conducted at Duke University Medical Center in North Carolina found that people with type 2 diabetes who scored higher on tests measuring their altruistic tendencies (or willingness to put others first) tended to have worse blood glucose control. However, people who had stronger tendencies to worry and experience other negative emotions such as anger, frustration, guilt, sadness, and hopelessness actually had better glucose control. One reason, researchers theorize, is that this latter group, with their higher levels of worrying, are more motivated to follow the kind of self-care needed to ensure good blood glucose outcomes.

Learning How to Breathe Again

Of all the things you might need to learn, how to breathe certainly wouldn't be on your list, right? But it's quite likely that you're not breathing correctly. Most people use less than half the capacity of their lungs in regular breathing, taking quick, shallow breaths that make the top part of their chests rise slightly. Because we breathe in and out an average of 21,000 times a day, that's a lot of missed opportunity.

On the other hand, deep breathing from your *diaphragm*—the lower part of your chest—can slow that cavalcade of stress hormones and help

MedLingo

The **diaphragm** is the muscular partition separating the abdominal and lung, or thoracic, cavities. It plays a central role in respiration. When the diaphragm is pulled down, the chest cavity expands. This reduces the pressure in the lungs so that outside air, which is at a higher pressure, moves into the lungs.

restore your body to homeostasis (remember that word from earlier in the book?) in just a couple of minutes.

After you have the routine down, you can call upon this stress-reduction technique any time you feel yourself shifting into fight-or-flight mode.

1. Put your hand over your stomach.

2. Close your eyes and (try to) empty your mind.

3. Take in a deep breath, but don't stop when you normally do. Instead, make sure you feel your hand rise.

4. Hold the breath in for a few seconds, and then slowly exhale.

5. Repeat 10 times.

Bet You Didn't Know

Deep breathing is so conducive to lowering blood pressure that the U.S. Food and Drug Administration actually approved a device designed to help you breathe better for just that purpose. Called the RespeRate, it is a paperback-book-size device that analyzes your breathing via a sensor buckled around your waist, and then plays musical tones to guide you through 15-minute breathing exercises to lower your breathing rate.

Meditating Your Stress Levels Away

If the thought of meditation brings to mind bald-headed men in orange robes chanting "Ohmmmm," you're behind the times. Today, meditation has been linked with so many positive health outcomes that it's taught in many medical schools and is a regular part of many cardiovascular rehabilitation programs to help people after a heart attack.

More recently, meditation has been used to help people with diabetes better control their disease. In one study, 108 people with type 2 diabetes received a five-session group diabetes education program. Part of the group received stress management training as part of the program, including meditation and mental imagery, whereas the others did not.

Those who received the stress management training had a 0.5 percent reduction in their HbA1c levels one year after the training ended. It might not sound like a lot, but even this modest change has been associated with a significant reduction (15-20 percent) in the risk of *microvascular* (or small vessel) *complications,* such as those that lead to blindness and kidney disease. Of course, you need to maintain this improvement to realize the beneficial effect on your risk for complications.

MedLingo

Microvascular compli-cations result from damage to the smallest blood vessels in your body, such as those found in the eyes, nerves, and kidneys.

Picturing Yourself on a Beach ...

One form of meditation you might want to try is called mental imagery. With this stress-management technique, you let your mind take a vacation.

The first step is to come up with an image of something that is soothing to you. It could be a picture of yourself soaking in a bubble bath, lying on a beach, or even skiing down a double-black diamond (hey, to each his own).

Now close your eyes and create the scene. If you're in the bath, for instance, feel the warmth of the water, smell the scent of the bubbles, see the flicker of candle flames against your eyes, hear the soothing quiet of the still bathroom, and feel yourself enveloped in a humid, warm cocoon.

Now open your eyes. Are you still as stressed out by disagreement you had with your boss over the new project?

You might also want to seek out training in guided mental imagery, in which you listen to tapes that guide you through a mental image designed to relax you.

> **Bet You Didn't Know**
>
> If you want to learn meditation, you really should take a class. Although it doesn't sound difficult in theory—sit in a quiet place, clear your mind, and focus on your breathing or a word for 5 to 10 minutes—it really does take some practice. You can find qualified practitioners through stress-reduction programs in your community.

Progressive Muscle Relaxation

This is another stress-management technique used in the Duke study mentioned earlier in this chapter. Progressive muscle relaxation is just what it sounds like: a technique in which you train yourself to tense and then relax each group of muscles.

In the beginning, you learn to relax individual muscles (such as your eyes, your neck, or your feet). After you've practiced this enough, you should get good enough to relax your entire body at once.

To start, sit in a chair or lie on the couch in a quiet room. Start with your toes. Curl your toes on your right foot tightly and hold for 10 seconds; then release and relax for 10 seconds. Now the left foot. Now, flex your right foot toward your face. Release. Now the left. Continue with each major group of muscles as you work your way up your body.

Don't grimace or tighten your face or other muscles when you're working on a muscle elsewhere. And don't forget to breathe; the relaxed, deep breathing described earlier comes in really handy here.

Focus on how the muscle feels when you're clenching it and then how it feels when you relax it. This is also a wonderful technique to practice if you're having trouble sleeping (more on sleep later in this chapter).

Do the entire sequence once a day if you can until you feel you are able to control your muscle tension. Be careful: if you have problems with pulled muscles, broken bones, or any other medical reason that prohibits you from exercising, consult your doctor first.

Yoga and Diabetes

An Indian practice, yoga's origins date back more than 5,000 years. Today, yoga has gone mainstream. Yoga studies have opened in even the smallest, most rural towns and it's hard to find a health club that doesn't offer one or more yoga classes.

The practice combines physical and breathing exercises with meditation, and has been shown in numerous studies to reduce levels of stress-related hormones. A few studies even suggest that it might help people with type 2 diabetes control their blood glucose levels.

Today, there are nearly as many types of yoga as there are ice-cream flavors, including high-intensity yoga programs that can help you lose weight. However, if stress control is what you're after, stick with the more traditional forms such as Hatha yoga.

Yoga classes generally cost between $8 and $10 a class, and can be found in freestanding yoga studios, YMCAs, gyms, and other exercise venues. Although there are no national standards or certifications for yoga teachers, you should look for one who has trained with a more experienced teacher and who continues to train. The teacher you choose should also have training in basic anatomy and the effects of yoga techniques on the body and should maintain yoga separate from religion.

Changing Your Attitude

Are you a glass-half-full or a glass-half-empty kind of person? If you're the latter, you will feel the effects of stress much more than someone who is the former.

That's because part of how our bodies react to stress depends on how we view it. If, for instance, you view a traffic jam as a *&^(%**# waste of your time, then you're more likely to release higher amounts of stress hormones—and subject your body to all their negative effects—than someone who views a traffic jam as a way to have a few minutes to him or herself, listen to a book on tape or, if traffic really isn't moving, pull out a magazine.

Now, it's quite likely that at this point in your life, your personality is pretty well set. You won't suddenly be able to change from a hard-charging, Type A kind of person into a mellow, pet-the-cat and listen-to-classical-music kind of person. But that doesn't mean you can't begin to change how you react to certain situations one at a time.

One way to do this is to make a list of the things in your life that most annoy you. You know, those things that lead to a tension headache, make you want to punch someone, and give you that tight feeling in your stomach and that ache in the back of your neck. Take that list and rank each item in order of annoyance. Now, take the top five to work on.

Let's say that the first one has to do with your boss. He's disorganized, unclear, and incapable of meeting deadlines. Instead of focusing only on his negatives, try to turn those into positives. For instance …

- His disorganization means that you, by comparison, look good.

- He's disorganized, yes, but he is very creative, which has resulted in some interesting projects for you.

- The fact that he can't meet deadlines means that you don't have to rush to meet them, either.

See? Each week, try to revise how you view one stressor. After you've worked your way through the first five, start on the second five. Keep going until the list is finished, by which time you'll probably have enough new stressors in your life to start a new list!

Getting Your Zzzzzzzssss

How'd you sleep last night? If you're like most Americans, not too well. Today, Americans get 25 percent less sleep than they did a century ago. Nearly four out of ten don't get the minimum seven hours of sleep necessary for optimal health and daytime functioning, while 15 percent get less than six hours most nights.

Such figures have only grown worse in recent years. Overall, nearly half (45 percent) of adults surveyed in a 2000 National Sleep Foundation poll say that they sleep less than eight hours to get more done for work, home, family, and hobbies.

> **Warning**
>
> Do you wake up hungry in the middle of the night? If you're taking insulin, make sure that you are also eating a small bedtime snack. If you are, then talk to your doctor about adjusting your evening dose of insulin. You might be suffering from nocturnal hypoglycemia, in other words, low blood sugar at night.

That's not only lousy for your health in general, but for your blood sugar in particular.

The links between sleep and blood sugar first surfaced in the late 1990s, when researchers at the University of Chicago found that depriving healthy young men of a good night's sleep raised their blood glucose levels nearly as high as those of people with diabetes. Later studies by the same group found that lack of sleep significantly increased insulin resistance in healthy adults, putting them at significant risk for the *metabolic syndrome*, a constellation of conditions that is often a precursor for diabetes and heart attacks.

> **MedLingo**
>
> A **syndrome** is usually defined as group of signs and symptoms that occur together and characterize a particular abnormality. The **metabolic syndrome**, however, is defined a bit differently. It refers to a constellation of conditions (rather than signs and symptoms) that includes obesity, insulin resistance, high blood pressure, high glucose levels, high triglyceride levels, and low HDL cholesterol (the "good" cholesterol). People with the metabolic syndrome are at increased risk for developing cardiovascular disease.

Another study, this one from Harvard Medical School, found that women who sleep five or fewer hours a day are nearly a third more likely to develop diabetes.

No one knows for sure just why too little sleep affects glucose levels, but there are some theories. One is that how much sleep you get, as well as the quality of that sleep, relates to your body's ability to control the release of various hormones. A few nights spent tossing and turning can cause that system to fall out of whack.

Note the word *quality* here. That is another link between diabetes and sleep that is better understood. People with diabetes, particularly those who tend to be overweight, and especially those who are obese, are more likely to have a condition known as *sleep-disordered breathing*, or SDB. The disorder, which includes *sleep apnea*, affects between 5 and 10 percent of middle-aged adults and 20 to 30 percent of the elderly. It significantly affects how well you sleep, even if you don't know it.

People with sleep apnea stop breathing for a couple of seconds many times during the night. You don't know you're not breathing, but your sleep is disrupted nonetheless because every time you stop breathing, your brain gets a signal to wake you up to start breathing again; so you don't get the deep, restful sleep you need.

Consequently, you feel tired, headachy, and sluggish the next day. The condition is also strongly associated with an increased risk for cardiovascular disease, high blood pressure, and heart attack. There's even some evidence that sleep apnea and other forms of SDB might increase the risk of developing diabetes.

If you already have diabetes, however, the question becomes whether the SDB is a result of your diabetes or the diabetes related to the SDB. No one really knows; one theory is that high blood sugar damages the part of the nervous system that controls breathing, and therefore plays a role in breathing problems during sleep. Another theory links the two to the obesity and being overweight, which is so common in people with diabetes.

We should have more answers in the future. In 2003, the National Institutes of Health announced it would fund a large clinical trial on the connection between the metabolic syndrome, which includes insulin resistance, and breathing-related sleep disorders.

Warning

If you're diagnosed with a sleep-related breathing disorder (or think you might have one), don't take sedatives or sleeping pills to help you snooze. They can keep you from waking up enough to begin breathing again when you stop.

Bet You Didn't Know

A lack of sleep can contribute to your weight problems. Studies find that levels of leptin, often known as the appetite hormone because low levels stimulate the appetite, are lower in people who are sleep deprived. This makes you hungrier, particularly for high-fat, high-carbohydrate foods.

Getting Evaluated for Sleep Disorders

If your partner has been complaining about your snoring, don't take it lightly. As someone with diabetes, you already have an increased risk for cardiovascular disease. Put a sleep-related breathing disorder on top of that and you're putting yourself in serious trouble.

Thankfully, doctors are getting pretty good at treating sleep apnea and other such disorders. Weight loss or even just learning to sleep on your side or stomach can help. If your condition is more severe, you may need nasal continuous positive airway pressure (CPAP), in which you wear a mask over your nose while you sleep. Pressure from an air blower forces air through your nasal passages, which prevents your airway from closing.

Dental devices are also available that reposition the lower jaw and tongue. Surgery might also be an option. Common surgical procedures for sleep-related breathing disorders include removing adenoids, tonsils, nasal polyps, other growths or tissue in the airway or surgery to correct structural deformities.

Sugar Sense

If your partner has been complaining about your snoring and you have a hard time sleeping on your stomach, try sewing a tennis ball onto the back of a pajama top or t-shirt that you sleep in. The tennis ball will keep you from sleeping on your back.

So talk to your doctor about your concerns. You need to be evaluated in a sleep disorders clinic. You spend the night in the clinic hooked up to sensors that record your brain waves and other physiological changes during the night, but this isn't as bad as it sounds. It might not be the best way to get a good night's sleep, but it could be a good way save your life in the future.

Getting a Good Night's Sleep

So, you're wondering, how can you keep from tossing and turning all night? Try these tried-and-true remedies:

- Make your bedroom a sleep-only haven. Remove clutter, get the computer and the TV out, and invest in some room-darkening curtains or shades.

- Use your bed for sleeping and before-bed reading (and sex) only.

- Take a hot bath at least two hours before you plan to go to bed. Any later, and your core temperature will be too high; cooler is always better when it comes to sleep.

- ◆ Avoid any caffeine, alcohol, or exercise in the three hours before you want to go to sleep.

- ◆ Put your alarm clock under your bed so you can't see the time.

- ◆ Try a soothing nighttime tea such as chamomile.

- ◆ Spray your pillow with the soothing scent of lavender, which is a known relaxant.

When You're Not Feeling Well

Your throat is scratchy, your joints are achy, and that headache that's been threatening all day has just come on like gangbusters. It's a virus and maybe even the flu. Before you know it, you're curled up in bed feeling like you've just been hit with a truck—twice.

As terrible as you feel, now is not the time to ignore your diabetes. When you're sick, your body is under considerable stress. As we already discussed, stress of any type can affect your blood sugar levels, increasing your liver's production of glucose while at the same time making your muscle cells more insulin resistant.

Plus, when you're sick, you're sometimes throwing up, have diarrhea, and often don't feel like eating or drinking—all of which throws your body chemistry out of whack and can lead to serious complications.

One of these complications is called *hyperosmolar-nonketotic coma*, also called *hyperglycemic nonketotic syndrome*. It literally means "coma due to thick blood." Although it can occur in people who don't know that they have diabetes or those with diabetes who have had high blood sugars for quite some time, it

MedLingo

Hyperosmolar-nonketotic coma, also called *hyperglycemic nonketotic syndrome*, is a form of very uncontrolled diabetes with extremely high blood glucose levels that occurs without the presence of ketones in your urine. It often occurs when you're ill and dehydrated. Common symptoms include weakness, severe thirst and increased urination, nausea, and lethargy.

Sugar Sense

If you're sick, you don't need to worry about any over-the-counter medications you're taking such as cough drops, cough syrup, and so on. Although there used to be some concern that the sugar they contain could affect blood glucose levels, studies find that's not the case. One less thing for you to worry about!

more commonly occurs during episodes of acute illness, particularly if you're severely dehydrated (hence the thick blood). It's also more common in elderly people.

Common symptoms include weakness, severe thirst and increased urination, nausea, and lethargy. Your blood sugar levels can rise as high as 1,000 mg/dl or even higher. Eventually confusion and coma result. These symptoms generally come on gradually, over several days. But they are a warning you should heed: about 25 percent of those who develop hyperosmolar-nonketotic coma die. This is more likely to happen in the elderly, however.

Caring for Yourself When You're Sick

One of the most important things to do when you're sick is to make sure you don't become dehydrated. If your blood sugar levels are already too high, your kidneys will pull excess fluid from your body, resulting in excessive urination and contributing to dehydration. To make sure you don't become dehydrated you've got to push the liquids.

MedLingo

Electrolytes are dissolved salts in your body that are very important in maintaining homeostasis.

Sugar Sense

If you were used to "powering through" an illness pre-diabetes, you've got to change. Now is the time to rest and take care of yourself and let someone else take care of you, too. Forget going into work, take a break from exercise, and cancel all commitments. Even something as simple as a cold can become very serious for someone with diabetes.

◆ Fill a gallon jug with ice and water and keep it by your bed. Make sure you drink at least 10 ounces of liquid every 30 minutes to an hour.

◆ If you're not very hungry, try clear soups or even Jell-O to keep some nutrients going in and maintain hydration. Clear soups (just dissolve a bouillon cube in boiling water) can also keep your *electrolytes* balanced with their high salt content.

◆ Suck on sugar-free popsicles.

Regardless of how you're feeling, you still need to take your medicine, whether that's insulin or oral medications. Let your doctor know if you're unable to eat or keep down any food; you might need to adjust your insulin dose. Also let your doctor know if you're vomiting up your oral medication.

Occasionally, your doctor might also start you on insulin, just temporarily, if your blood sugar levels remain very high for more than several days.

However, this isn't easy. You'll have to be admitted to the hospital while you learn how to use insulin and the results are monitored.

Speaking of blood sugar levels: you need to keep checking your blood sugar every three to four hours. If you don't feel up to it, get someone else in the house to test for you. Make sure they know what they're looking for: if you notice either a major spike (most meters will read this as "critically high" or use a similar term), or consistent levels above 300 mg/dl, you might be heading into hyperosmolar-nonketotic coma.

Also check your urine for the presence of ketones if you can. Although it's rare in people with type 2 diabetes, you do have a slight chance of diabetic ketoacidosis when you're sick. You can buy ketone strips at the drugstore.

The Least You Need to Know

♦ Stress can significantly affect your blood sugar levels.

♦ Stress management techniques such as meditation, mental imagery, and deep breathing can help you better manage the stress in your life and your blood sugar levels.

♦ The quantity and quality of the sleep you get can affect your blood sugar levels.

♦ When you're sick, it's critical that you take good care of yourself, prevent dehydration, and rest.

What About Sex?

In This Chapter

- Your sex life on diabetes
- Erectile dysfunction and diabetes
- The little blue pill and beyond
- Women, diabetes, and desire
- Treatments for women few and far between

We told you earlier that diabetes affects every part of your life. Well, your sexual life is no exception. As far back as the first century, doctors connected sexual problems with diabetes. The writer of a medical encyclopedia of that time noted the "collapse of sexual function" as a specific complication of the disease. Even before any official studies, researchers declared in 1906 that impotence was one of the most common symptoms of diabetes.

If there ever was a good time to have this problem, however, today is it. With new medications on the market for men, and a growing body of research exploring women's sexuality, there is more help and support available than ever before.

Starting with the Men

We're going to start with the men, not because they're more important, but because they're better studied. We simply know more about sexual dysfunction in men with diabetes than we do in women. We also have more tried-and-true treatments.

MedLingo

Erectile dysfunction, also called **impotence,** refers to a man's inability to have and/or maintain an erection.

The sad fact is that if you have diabetes, you're more likely to experience *erectile dysfunction* (ED), or *impotence,* defined as the inability to have and maintain an erection, and to experience it earlier in your life than a man who doesn't have diabetes. In fact, studies find the risk of ED in men with type 2 diabetes is about twice as high as that of men without diabetes (it's three times more likely in men with type 1 diabetes, however).

Overall, estimates are that between 35 to 75 percent of men with diabetes will experience ED, with some studies finding that more than half of men with diabetes will experience ED within 10 years of their diagnosis. Compare that to overall rates of impotence, which affect about 5 percent of 40-year-old men and between 15 and 25 percent of 65-year-old men.

Studies also find that the longer you've had diabetes, the worse your glucose management, and the more complications you have, the more likely you are to experience ED.

Impotence and ED have received a lot of press in the past few years, ever since the Food and Drug Administration approved the sale of a little blue pill called Viagra (sildenafil) in March 1998 to treat the condition.

Almost overnight, it seemed, reports of ED in men (with and without diabetes) skyrocketed. In 1985, about 7.7 physician visits out of every 1,000 (for men) were regarding ED; in 1999, that figure shot up to 22.3 per 1,000 visits. Did more men suddenly find themselves impotent? Of course not. But now that there was an easy-to-take treatment, more men were willing to talk to their doctors about the problem (all those television ads about the ED didn't hurt, either).

Anatomy of an Erection

Before we talk about how diabetes affects erections, it's important to understand exactly how an erection occurs.

It starts, as you probably know, with either mental or physical stimulation. This in turn, sends signals to your brain, which then tells the nerve endings in the penis to release a chemical, called *nitric oxide*.

Nitric oxide relaxes or dilates blood vessels, enabling them to open up and bring more blood to the penis, swelling the penile tissues and helping to create an erection. At the same time, the dilated blood vessels that go into the penis press up against the blood vessels leaving the penis. This also helps to create an erection because it traps increased blood in the penis.

So three things have to work normally for a man to get an erection once he gets sexually excited:

- The nerves going into the penis

- Increased blood flow into the penis

- Trapping of that increased blood in the penis

MedLingo _____

Nitric oxide is a chemical that, among its many functions, relaxes blood vessels. It plays a role in erections by enabling more blood to flow into the penis to create an erection.

Once an orgasm occurs, the constriction of the blood vessels leaving the penis is relieved, the extra blood leaves, and the penis becomes soft again.

Diabetes, however, can play havoc with this chain of events in oh-so-many ways.

- **Nerve damage.** A common complication of diabetes resulting from poor blood sugar control, damage to the nerves in the penis can interfere with their ability to receive signals from the brain.

- **Vascular damage.** Sometimes there is a build-up of *plaque*, called *atherosclerosis* (we discuss this more in Chapter 16) in the arteries that feed blood into the penis. If it's bad enough, those vessels become partially blocked, preventing enough blood from getting into the penis.

MedLingo _____

Atherosclerosis occurs when **plaque**, a substance composed of cholesterol, fibrous tissue, blood components, and calcium, builds up on the walls of arteries, stiffening and narrowing the arteries and interfering with arterial function and blood flow.

Hypertension refers to blood pressure levels 140/90 or higher.

◆ **Heart disease and** *hypertension.* Both are common complications of diabetes, and some medications for both can play a role in ED. This risk for ED is higher in men with diabetes than in men without.

It Might Not Be Your Diabetes' Fault

Having said all that, we want to make something clear: Your diabetes may not be the reason for your ED. That's why you should talk to your doctor about any sexual problems.

MedLingo _____

Testosterone is the major sex hormone in men. It contributes to a man's sexual desire and influences his ability to have an erection.

MedLingo _____

Creatinine is a breakdown product of an amino acid (called creatine) that is part of muscles. It is eliminated in the urine. When the kidneys start to fail, it backs up into the blood. So high levels of blood creatinine mean kidney problems.

Other factors at play include psychological problems like depression, stress, anxiety, medications, or low *testosterone* levels due to something else besides diabetes, such as obesity.

Testing, Testing, Testing

After conducting a complete physical examination and medical history, your doctor may want to run some tests to get at the probable cause of your ED. These include blood counts, urinalysis, cholesterol and triglyceride levels, and measurements of *creatinine* (a marker for kidney health) and liver enzymes (to check the health of your liver).

Additionally, your doctor will probably want to measure the amount of testosterone in your blood, which can provide clues about any problems with your endocrine system.

Frankly, if you complain of ED, most physicians will probably just give you the "little blue pill" or one of its cousins unless there is a reason not to. Some doctors, however, may want to run other tests, including the following:

◆ *Nocturnal penile tumescence test.* Also called the stamp test, or the rigidity test, this test is conducted to see if you're having erections during the night while sleeping. Men normally have three to five involuntary erections at night. If you're having any, you most likely have a psychological cause for your ED vs. a physical cause. Your doctor may have you do the test at home or in a sleep laboratory. Generally, you put a ringlike device called a "snap gauge" around your penis. It is composed of plastic films that break at various pressures. If you have an erection, the film will be broken in the morning.

Bet You Didn't Know

Contrary to popular belief, ED is not an unavoidable consequence of getting older. Rather, in most instances ED is the result of some physical illness. In fact, diabetes, kidney disease, chronic alcoholism, multiple sclerosis, atherosclerosis, and neurologic diseases account for about 70 percent of all cases of ED. Additionally, numerous medications can affect a man's ability to have and maintain an erection. These include antihypertensives, antidepressants, antihistamines, tranquilizers, appetite suppressants, and cimetidine (an ulcer drug).

Or your doctor can use an electronic monitoring device that fits on your penis and provides information about how many erections you have, how long they lasted, and how intense they were.

◆ *Intracavernosal injection test.* This is a more invasive and uncomfortable test involving the injection of a medication, usually the hormone prostaglandin E., into the base of your penis. This medication typically produces an erection if you have no physical problems. Another way to get this drug into the penis is through a suppository inserted into the *urethra*, the tube through which urine leaves the penis. The doctor then measures how full and stiff your erection is, and how long it lasts. As you can tell, this test isn't much fun and is rarely performed any more.

The Little Blue Pill and Beyond

The good news, as we mentioned earlier, is that there are several treatments available today for ED. The bad news is that if you are taking a certain medication for heart disease, called a nitrate, your options may be limited. Let's start with the pills.

Today, there are three oral medications approved for the treatment of ED in men. These medications, Viagra (sildenafil), Levitra (vardenafil), and Cialis (tadalafil), belong to a class of drugs called PDE$_5$ inhibitors.

These drugs prevent the enzyme that normally breaks down nitric oxide from doing its job. That in turn, keeps more nitric oxide around longer. The biggest difference between the three is in how long they remain active and how long before intercourse you need to take them.

These drugs are not wonder drugs, however. They work only if you are sexually stimulated. They won't increase your *libido*, or your desire to have sex, only your ability.

All have similar side effects, including flushing, headache, heartburn, and sinus congestion, and you shouldn't take any if you're also taking a medication containing nitrates, often prescribed for heart disease.

You also shouldn't take them with an illegal drug called "poppers," which also contains nitrates and which is often used to enhance sexual pleasure. Together, the combination could cause your blood pressure to drop dangerously low, possibly leading to a heart attack or stroke.

Also, if you are taking a certain medication for hypertension or an enlarged prostate called an *alpha blocker*, you should not take Viagra and the alpha blocker within four hours of each other. Doing so could result in a dangerous drop in blood pressure. Check with your doctor to see if you are on an alpha blocker.

MedLingo

Libido refers to the desire to have sex.

Alpha blockers are medications used to treat hypertension and an enlarged prostate.

Five years of studies find that all heart patients except those taking nitrates can use Viagra safely. Levitra and Cialis haven't been on the market long enough to know if this applies to them, also.

Most studies find that the medications work pretty well in men with diabetes, although not as well as they work in men without the disease. Don't get frustrated if one doesn't work for you, however. Ask your doctor to try another. Cialis, for instance, appears to be more effective than Viagra, and might be a better option if the little blue pill doesn't work.

Viagra: The Pill That Started It All

Of the millions of words that have been written about Viagra since its introduction in 1998, perhaps nothing captures its intense popularity as much as this little statistic, courtesy of Viagra manufacturer Pfizer, Inc.: Nine Viagra tablets are dispensed *every second* worldwide. Wow!

Once taken, Viagra can work in as quickly as 30 minutes, but it may take longer in some men. Therefore, you should take it at least 30 minutes or more before having sex. It works for about four hours. You should take it only once a day, however.

One rare side effect from Viagra is temporary changes in your color vision (such as trouble telling the difference between blue and green objects), or objects having a blue tinge. This usually goes away in a few hours, however.

One other rare side effect is *priapism*, the presence of a persistent, usually painful, erection of the penis. When it occurs, it is usually after sex. If this lasts for four to six hours, and especially if it becomes painful, you should go to an emergency room. Priapism can result in damage to the penis and requires treatment.

Most studies suggest that Viagra works fairly well in men with diabetes, although one large study of 282 men conducted in Iran found that that number of erections was lower, and the rate of cardiovascular side effects higher in men with diabetes than reported in similar studies in men without diabetes.

Warning

Skip the high-fat hamburger and fries before taking Viagra or Levitra. Consuming a heavy meal may slow the drug's effect, meaning it will take longer before you can have an erection.

Loving with Levitra

Levitra, approved by the FDA in August 2003, works similarly to Viagra. Package instructions call for it to be taken an hour before you plan to have sex, but a 2004 study found that it began working in as little as 10 minutes and remained effective up to 12 hours.

About the only advantage of Levitra over Viagra is that it doesn't have the color vision side effect.

Cialis: Last out of the Gate but Gaining Fast

Cialis was approved for the treatment of ED in November 2003. It is just as effective as Viagra in comparative studies, but may be more effective in men with diabetes who have hard-to-treat ED.

Another advantage of Cialis is that it works within 30 minutes, and one dose remains effective up to 36 hours—far longer than the other two ED medications. Like the others, however, you shouldn't take Cialis if you're taking any kind of nitrate or alpha blocker. Also, food doesn't seem to affect how fast or how well Cialis works.

Beyond the Pills

If you can't take one of the PDE_5 inhibitors, or they aren't working for you, don't despair; there are other options. These include the following:

- **Testosterone.** Available in a patch or as an injection every two to three weeks, additional testosterone might be effective in restoring erections in men with low testosterone levels.

- **Other drugs.** Alprostadil is a drug approved for the treatment of ED. It comes in two forms: One is injected into the side of the penis (Caverject), while the other is a suppository that is inserted into the urethra. Unfortunately, the shot appears to be most effective, with success rates approaching 85 percent. The most common side effect is a burning sensation in the penis and persistent erection, or priapism, as discussed earlier. Since the success of the PDE$_5$ inhibitors, this treatment is used less often.

- **External devices.** If you don't want to take medication, you can try something called a vacuum constriction device. You slip a relatively large plastic tube with a band around the bottom over the penis, pushing it firmly over the skin at the base.

  You then use an attached pump to create a vacuum. This suction draws blood into the penis, resulting in an erection. The band around the bottom of the tube is slipped down around the base of the penis trapping the blood and maintaining the erection.

  The tube is removed and, voilà! You're ready to go. It's not very spontaneous, but it is very effective. The band should be released in 30 to 60 minutes.

- **Surgery.** Used only in the most extreme cases of ED, surgical procedures involve placing an implant into the penis to restore erection. This procedure is rarely used anymore because of potential complications.

Sexual Dysfunction: Women Get It, Too

The research into sexual functioning in women with diabetes lags far behind that of men. So far behind, in fact, that a 2003 article reviewing the medical literature on the topic published found only 25 published articles on the issue of female sexual function and diabetes.

That's not too surprising because research into women's sexual functioning overall lags far behind that of men. There are many reasons, including the fact that it's just more difficult to study women's sexuality. After all, it's pretty easy to measure an erection; it's not as simple to tell if a woman is sexually stimulated or satisfied.

However, this lack of interest is beginning to change. The impetus for increased research activity into women's sexual function comes from two sources: the popularity of Viagra, and a 1999 article published in the *Journal of the American Medical Association* (JAMA). The article reported on a survey of 1,749 women and 1,410 men, finding that 43 percent of the women reported some form of sexual dysfunction compared to 31 percent of the men.

Given that studies on the effect of diabetes on women's sexuality are few and far between, what we're about to say here must be taken with the proverbial grain of salt. We'll let you know what those few studies found, and then focus primarily on what you can do if you're having sexual problems, whether or not they're related to your diabetes.

Numbers Vary

The amount of sexual problems among women with diabetes remains a hazy number. Some studies show no differences in sexual dysfunction between women with and without the disease, while others show significant differences, particularly for women with type 2 diabetes. In fact, one 1983 study found that women with type 2 diabetes were more likely to have sexual problems than women with type 1.

The author concluded, however, that this might be due to the fact that women are typically diagnosed with type 2 at a later age, usually after menopause, and when they're overweight, each of which is a risk factor for sexual problems on its own.

Overall, though, it does appear that women with diabetes are more likely to experience sexual problems than women without. One important study found that while 47 percent of participating women with diabetes reported sexual dysfunction, 89 percent said their problems started *after* their diabetes diagnosis.

The most commonly reported problems are the following:

- ◆ Decrease in sexual desire
- ◆ Decrease in sexual arousal or lubrication
- ◆ Pain during intercourse
- ◆ Problems with orgasm

So What's Going On?

Although we have a fairly good idea about the diabetes-related causes of sexual problems in men, the connection in women remains fairly murky. What is clear is that the problems are not limited to physical changes caused by the diabetes or to complications.

In one large study of women with type 1 diabetes, for instance, researchers found that sexual dysfunction was related to dissatisfaction with their marriage, poor understanding of their diabetes, poor emotional adjustment to their diabetes, higher impact of their diabetes treatment on their daily life, and dissatisfaction with their treatment.

The women who were depressed also reported more sexual dysfunction, whereas those who weren't depressed reported no more sexual problems than did women without diabetes. Overall, the researchers concluded, sexual dysfunction in women with diabetes seems to be more related to psychological than physical problems.

Although this study was conducted in women with type 1 diabetes, the results would, quite likely, be the same for women with type 2 diabetes, especially for women taking insulin.

A key component seems to be acceptance of your disease. After you accept the reality of your diabetes and the treatment required, the researchers suggest, your sexual functioning should improve. Another key component is satisfaction with your relationship.

All of which is not to say that the disease itself doesn't have some effect on overall sexuality. If your blood sugar is too high, for instance, you get very thirsty, right? Well, the same physical effects making you thirsty also dry out other tissues, including vaginal tissue.

Bet You Didn't Know

Marital satisfaction plays a major role in the health of those with diabetes above and beyond sexual health. Studies find that men with diabetes don't care for themselves as well if they have marital conflicts. They find that the more strongly your spouse believes in good blood glucose control, the more likely you are to control your glucose levels, and that the better the overall quality of your marriage, the better you'll adjust emotionally to your disease.

Bottom line is that the attention you pay to the health of your relationship is just as important as the attention you pay to your own physical health.

Additionally, as we talked about earlier in the book, women with diabetes and poorly controlled blood sugars are more likely to get vaginal yeast infections—certainly not conducive to feeling sexual.

Plus, if your blood sugar is under good control, you're just going to feel better overall. With a better mood, more energy, maybe even some weight loss because you're managing your disease better, you're more likely to feel sexy.

Treating the Problem: Few Options

Although more than a dozen drug manufacturers are rushing to be the first to bring a drug for female sexual dysfunction to market, to date their efforts have been disappointing. Even the manufacturers of Viagra gave up trying to see if the drug would work in women.

The problem is that women's sexuality is related to so many things other than blood flow. The quality of the relationship, the stress in the rest of her life, her own past sexual experiences, her physical health—all impact a woman's desire.

Having said that, there are a few medical options available for women with low sexual desire and/or sexual problems, all of which should be safe for women with diabetes (but, as always, check with your doctor). Among them are the following:

- **Supplemental testosterone.** Women make a small amount of testosterone (just as men make a small amount of estrogen), and the hormone plays a major role in their sexual desire. In 2004, an FDA committee rejected a testosterone patch designed to restore sexual desire in women who have undergone hysterectomies during menopause, saying the patch needed more study.

  But some doctors have been prescribing testosterone *off label* to women with sexual problems for years. Just make sure you understand the potential downside: increased hair growth the most common. Other potential side effects (particularly if the dose is too high) include deepening of the voice, acne, and, in spite of more hair on other parts of your body, loss of scalp hair in a pattern similar to men (called male-pattern baldness).

- **Eros Clitoral Therapy Device.** This FDA-approved device is available by prescription only. It is a small, handheld device that is placed over the *clitoris* to create a gentle vacuum, increasing blood flow to the genital area.

MedLingo

Off-label use is when doctors prescribe an FDA-approved drug for something the drug is not officially approved for. The FDA only approves drugs for specific conditions that the drug has been tested in. However, once a drug has been approved for any indication, doctors are allowed to prescribe it for other conditions if they think that it will be helpful. Only if the FDA says that it is contra-indicated for a specific condition are doctors not supposed to prescribe it in that situation.)

Clitoris is a female sexual organ, similar to the penis.

◆ **Hormone therapy.** Several forms of estrogen, including creams and suppositories, are approved for the treatment of vaginal dryness and other vaginal symptoms associated with menopause that result in sexual problems. Talk to your doctor about whether this might be a good option for you.

◆ **Vaginal gels, creams, and suppositories.** These products, generally available over-the-counter, can counter any vaginal dryness, reducing pain during sex and making intercourse more pleasurable.

Beyond Medical Treatment

Studies find that a woman's self-image strongly affects how sexual she feels. Given that the health of a woman's relationship and her stress levels also play major roles in her sexual desire, it's important that women take a holistic approach to dealing with any sexual issues.

Sugar Sense

So let's assume for a minute that you have no sexual problems. Sex is great. You love it, and you have it a lot. What does that mean in terms of your blood sugar control? Well, sex *is* a physical activity. Thus, if you're taking insulin, it could cause low blood sugar levels. So consider a snack just before or after lovemaking.

That includes focusing on your own self-image and health. If you are overweight, for instance, you may not feel sexy (not to mention the way it may affect your blood glucose control).

If that's not an incentive to lose weight, we don't know what is! One of the best things we can recommend in terms of weight loss and improving your body image (and sex life) is regular exercise. Not only will it help with your weight, but it will also reduce stress, make you feel better about yourself (because you'll see what you can accomplish), and reduce your risk of depression.

You also need to work on your relationship if you're having problems (assuming you want to remain in the relationship). You might consider professional counseling. Or maybe the two of you simply need to refocus on each other. Regular dates, finding a new hobby you can do together, and sexual experimentation can all restore the luster to a dull relationship.

Because depression is often related to a lack of sexual desire, it's important to talk to your doctor about your mood. If you are depressed, then counseling, medication, or a combination of the two can make a huge difference in your overall mood—and libido.

The Least You Need to Know

- Men with diabetes are much more likely to experience erectile dysfunction (impotence) than men without diabetes.

- There are three oral medications and several other treatments available to treat impotence in men.

- Women with diabetes are more likely to have sexual dysfunction than women without diabetes.

- Women's sexual dysfunction is related primarily to emotional health and to how well they accept their disease.

- There are few medical treatments for women's sexual dysfunction, although emotional counseling and lifestyle changes may help.

Chapter 14

And Baby Makes Two

In This Chapter

- ◆ Planning your pregnancy
- ◆ Your pregnancy team
- ◆ Eating and exercising for two
- ◆ Labor and delivery

So you're thinking about having a baby, are you? Congratulations! That's a big step in so many ways: emotionally, financially, and physically. No, we're not talking about the weight gain and big belly. As someone with type 2 diabetes, you and your doctor are going to have many more worries when it comes to your health and the health of the baby than most pregnant women.

Hopefully you're reading this chapter before you've become pregnant, because the time to begin planning for this pregnancy begins right now—not the day the pregnancy test is positive. You have some serious getting ready to do if you want to ensure a healthy pregnancy and, most important, a healthy baby.

Behind the Blue and Pink: Facts About Pregnancy and Diabetes

You learned in Chapter 1 about a type of diabetes that occurs only in pregnancy called gestational diabetes. We're not going to deal with that type in this chapter. This chapter is devoted entirely to pregnancy, labor, and delivery in women already diagnosed with type 2 diabetes, whether you're on insulin, on oral drugs, or managing your disease with diet and exercise alone.

You should know that you're kind of unique. Until fairly recently, most pregnant women with diabetes had type 1 diabetes. That's because young, fertile women didn't get type 2 very often. Of course, as you saw in Chapter 1, that's changing. Today, although the overall prevalence, or occurrence, of diabetes increased 33 percent in the United States from 1990 to 1998 overall, the prevalence in people aged 30 to 39 increased by 70 percent!

That's translated into more pregnant women today with type 2 diabetes than with type 1 diabetes. And with adolescent rates of diabetes on the rise, experts are particularly concerned about the potential for dangers to the young girls and their fetuses from undiagnosed or undertreated diabetes if they accidentally get pregnant.

Here's the bottom line. Doctors are rapidly becoming aware that type 2 diabetes poses just as significant a risk to mother and baby as type 1 if you start with high or uncontrolled blood sugars and don't control them well during the pregnancy. We're not trying to scare you here; we just want you to understand the potential risks—and what you can do to minimize them.

Preventing Unplanned Pregnancies

As a woman with type 2 diabetes, it is critical that you do not become pregnant accidentally. That's because by the time you realize you're pregnant, you could be four or six weeks along. That might not sound like much in real-world time, but in developing-baby time, it's major. By the time that stick turns blue, many of your baby's major organs have formed. If your blood sugar levels are high, that could cause a problem with the baby's initial development.

The best way not to get pregnant (beyond abstaining from sex, of course) is good birth control. There's no reason you can't use oral contraceptives, diaphragms, IUDs, or any other contraceptive device. You might even want to talk to your doctor about a birth control device that is implanted in your arm, or a shot you get every three months; that way, you don't have to remember to take something every day as with birth control pills.

Unfortunately, too many women with diabetes get pregnant unintentionally, with one survey finding that figure as high as 60 percent.

Understanding the Risks

Although we're just now beginning to see large studies on pregnancies and their outcomes in women with type 2, what we're learning is pretty serious. It seems that type 2 diabetes carries just as many risks for mother and baby—maybe even more—than type 1 diabetes. Specifically, these include the following:

♦ High rates of preeclampsia. This is a dangerous condition in which a woman's blood pressure gets very high, she retains fluid, and she begins leaking protein into her urine, a sign of kidney problems. It can lead to eclampsia, a toxic condition in which the mother goes into convulsions and possibly a coma during or immediately after pregnancy. It puts both mother and baby's lives in jeopardy. In one study of 207 women with type 2 diabetes, nearly 40 percent developed preeclampsia—a rate even higher than in women with type 1 diabetes.

♦ High rates of miscarriage and stillbirths. Women with type 2 diabetes are about four times more likely to miscarry than women with type 1 diabetes, and nine times more likely to miscarry than women without diabetes.

♦ High rates of birth defects. The babies of women with type 2 diabetes are about five times more likely to have major birth defects, usually affecting the heart, central nervous system, or musculoskeletal system, than women without diabetes. This is particularly true if their mothers didn't follow a preconception diabetes program like the one we're going to talk about in a minute, resulting in out-of-control blood sugars when they became pregnant.

♦ Bigger babies. If your blood sugar is too high, your fetus gets too much glucose. This causes fat to build up around their shoulders and body, which could make them difficult to deliver vaginally, resulting in an early delivery or Cesarean section.

These higher rates of miscarriage, stillbirth, and birth defects are clearly connected with poorer control of a women's diabetes, both before and during the pregnancy.

For instance, in one study, women with HbA1c values less than 9.3 percent had a miscarriage rate of 12.4 percent, and a rate of major birth defects in their babies of 3 percent; women with HbA1c values of 14.4 percent or more had a 37.5 percent rate of miscarriage and 40 percent of their babies had major birth defects. Big difference, huh? This study included women with both types of diabetes.

And, it turns out, it doesn't matter whether you're taking insulin, oral medications, or managing your diabetes with lifestyle changes during your pregnancy—if you have hyperglycemia, your child has an increased risk of problems.

But pregnancy and birth-related complications in women with type 2 diabetes are also related to factors beyond blood sugar control. Women with type 2 diabetes are likely to be older and overweight when they get pregnant, and have high blood pressure.

Bet You Didn't Know

There's some thought that diabetes during pregnancy may play a role in the increasing rates of diabetes among children, because infants are exposed to diabetes while in the womb. This, in turn, is thought to lead to a condition called *fetal hyperinsulinemia*, in which the fetus has too much insulin in his or her blood. This increases the number of fat cells in the infant, resulting in obesity and insulin resistance in childhood.

Insulin Resistance

Pregnancy itself causes insulin resistance in all women, whether they have diabetes or not. This is because the *placenta* produces its own hormones, some of which interfere with the action of insulin. Because the placenta gets bigger as the baby grows, insulin resistance increases throughout pregnancy.

MedLingo

The **placenta** is a temporary organ that connects a mother with her growing fetus and allows for the transfer of nutrients and other materials to pass from mother to baby.

The plus side to this insulin resistance? It means there are low rates of hypoglycemia in pregnant women with type 2 diabetes, making tight blood sugar control easier from at least one perspective.

Now, don't freak out! Just because you have diabetes doesn't mean you can't have a healthy pregnancy and baby—it's just going to take some preparation and work.

Planning for Your Pregnancy

Why is it so important to plan your pregnancy? There are so many reasons!

- ◆ You're much more likely to see an obstetrician before you become pregnant if you plan the pregnancy.

- ◆ Your risk of complications during the pregnancy or delivery, or of problems with the baby, decrease significantly.

- ◆ You will receive more supportive and positive feedback from your medical team while you're trying to become pregnant and during your pregnancy.

- ◆ You can ensure that you are in the best possible health before you get pregnant, from controlled blood sugars to a healthy weight to starting on prenatal vitamins.

Ideally, you should start your preconception planning three to six months before you want to start getting pregnant.

Centralizing Your Care

The first step in planning for your pregnancy is finding the right doctor. Although you've probably been doing really well with your primary-care physician, maybe with a visit to the endocrinologist every few months, you need an obstetrician on your side, preferably one who specializes in *high-risk* pregnancies like yours.

These doctors, also called *perinatologists*, are a kind of super-charged ob/gyn. They've had additional training in the pregnancies and their pregnancy and delivery. Often affiliated with major academic medical centers, they practice in hospitals that have special nurseries to take care of very sick babies.

But don't think you're turning your back on your primary-care doctor for nine months! Oh no. Your regular doctor still needs to stay in the picture and work closely with your ob/gyn *and* your existing endocrinologist. You'll still need help from your diabetes educator and dietitian

MedLingo

A **high-risk** pregnancy is one in which the mother and/or fetus has some underlying condition or problem that puts one or both of them at risk for complications. Specially trained physicians, called **perinatologists**, generally treat women with high-risk pregnancies. A **neonatologist** is a doctor specially trained to take care of very sick newborns.

(now more than ever), and, possibly, a social worker. As your pregnancy progresses, you will add a pediatrician or *neonatologist*, a pediatrician specially trained to take care of very sick newborns, to your team.

Expect to see your doctors—all of them—fairly often during your pregnancy, certainly more often than a pregnant woman who doesn't have diabetes.

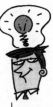

Sugar Sense _____

Make sure you start taking a prenatal vitamin about three months before you get pregnant. Studies find that the B vitamin *folic acid* is critical in preventing certain birth defects like *spina bifida* in infants, and that the first few weeks of pregnancy (often before you even know you're pregnant) is the most critical time.

But don't forget—you are the core of your team. You call the shots, and if someone suggests something that makes you feel uncomfortable, speak up! On the other hand, your healthcare team can only suggest what you should do. You have the final say whether it gets done or not. Remember: you are responsible not only for your own health, but also for your baby's. That's a lot of responsibility!

The Goals of Preconception Care

The goal of your preconception program is to get your HbA1c values as close to normal as possible (in most labs this is 6 percent or less.) Ideally, you should maintain values less than 1 percent above normal. The lower your HbA1c levels, the lower your risk for miscarriage and birth defects in the baby.

MedLingo _____

Folic acid is a B vitamin critical in the healthy development of a fetus.

Spina bifida is a birth defect in which the fetal spine fails to fuse early in development.

How do you get there? Well, by now you should know the drill:

- ◆ Follow a good meal plan.

- ◆ Monitor your blood glucose levels on a regular basis.

- ◆ Continue taking your medications or insulin as needed (and adjusting insulin dosages as necessary to maintain good blood control).

- Treat any episodes of hypoglycemia immediately.

- Get regular exercise.

- Reduce your stress level and learn to better cope with the stress you do have.

Piece of cake, right?

Getting Started

So you've got your pregnancy medical team in place; great. Make an appointment with your new obstetrician for a pre-pregnancy evaluation. This should include a complete medical history, physical examination for any diabetes-related complications, and various and sundry laboratory tests.

At this time, if you're taking oral glucose medications, your doctor will talk to you about insulin. Once you get pregnant, you'll likely immediately switch from oral meds to insulin. Don't panic! It doesn't mean that your diabetes has gotten worse. It's just that the oral medications could affect the baby; plus, as we noted earlier, you're going to become much more insulin resistant once you become pregnant; the additional insulin will come in handy.

> **Bet You Didn't Know**
>
> You might be able to stay on your medication if you're taking the sulfonylurea drug glyburide. Studies on women with gestational diabetes found no difference in terms of blood glucose or numbers of abnormally large infants between women who used glyburide or insulin, and found no evidence of the drug in the baby's cord blood (a sign that it didn't cross the placenta into the baby).

Make sure your doctor knows about every drug you're taking, even over-the-counter medications. Many medications can harm the developing baby, sometimes even before you know for sure you're pregnant.

One that people with diabetes often take and that we know can cause birth defects is an ACE inhibitor. This medication is often taken to treat high blood pressure, or early kidney disease. The trouble occurs in the first trimester, so make sure you stop taking it before you become pregnant (with your doctor's approval, of course).

When the Stick Turns Blue

So you started your preconception program and, after three months, buried your last pack of birth control pills in the back yard and settled into trying to get pregnant.

A few months later, you missed your period, threw up after smelling the morning coffee, and bingo! You're pregnant.

Congratulations. Now the fun really begins!

First, because you're probably now taking insulin, you need to test your blood sugar at least three times a day, probably more. If you're not used to insulin, go back to Chapter 8 and review.

Next, you have to get used to checking your ketone levels every morning before you eat and before you take insulin. If you have ketones in your urine in even tiny amounts for two consecutive days, call your doctor! There's a chance you might have developed a condition called *starvation ketosis*, which means your muscle and other cells were so starved for glucose that your body began breaking down fat cells for energy, releasing ketones. This isn't dangerous to you but several studies find that babies from mothers who had high ketones during pregnancy had a slightly lower I.Q. when tested at ages four to five than children whose mothers avoided high ketone levels during pregnancy.

Starvation ketosis is easy to fix. All you have to do is eat more carbohydrates. Here's why.

It turns out that in pregnant women, glucose is released into the urine at lower blood glucose levels than before pregnancy. Thus, muscle and other cells can become starved for glucose because all that sugar gets lost into the urine instead of providing energy for muscles.

So your body has to start using more fat for energy. By eating more carbohydrates, more glucose becomes available for muscle to use and you can avoid ketosis.

> **MedLingo** _____
>
> **Starvation ketosis** occurs when your body begins breaking down fat for energy when there is not enough glucose to provide energy to muscle and other cells.

> **MedLingo** _____
>
> An **electrocardiogram (EKG or ECG)** measures and records your heart's electrical activity. During an EKG, electrodes are attached to your chest and, sometimes, your arms and legs. They detect your heart's electrical signals and send this information by wires, called leads, to a recording machine.

Your First Visit

During your first prenatal visit, your ob/gyn will take a complete medical history, weigh and measure you, and perform a battery of blood tests. So far, no different from a pregnant woman who doesn't have diabetes. Because you have diabetes, however, you'll get a few extra tests:

◆ A urine test to see if you have kidney damage. This could either be a 24-hour urine collection to test for albumin and creatinine or simply an early morning urine sample to measure the same two things.

◆ A blood test to test for creatinine

◆ An *electrocardiogram (EKG)* to test your heart function

Bet You Didn't Know

When you're pregnant, you're more likely to experience retinopathy, changes to tiny blood vessels in the eye. We'll talk more about retinopathy in Chapter 17, but you should know that pregnancy can make any existing retinopathy worse. That's why it's so important that you see an ophthalmologist for a full eye exam (preferably one who specializes in diseases of the retina, the back part of the eye where damage occurs due to diabetes) before you try to get pregnant. If you have retinopathy and it has gotten to the point where it needs treatment, you may be able to receive laser treatment to correct it before you become pregnant. Also make sure you continue to see your ophthalmologist two or three times during your pregnancy to make sure retinopathy hasn't developed, or that any existing retinopathy hasn't gotten worse.

Eating for Two

It's important to have a long talk with your dietitian about your nutritional needs during your pregnancy, and how that will be correlated with your body's increasing need for calories as your baby grows. He or she will work closely with you to go over your specific diet. What follows are some general principles.

First, you don't want to gain all your weight at once during your pregnancy. Instead, you should see the pounds come on gradually. (Enjoy this time; it's the only time in your life when a scale inching upward is a *good* thing.)

During the first trimester, for instance, you should gain a total of 2 to 5 pounds, while during the last two trimesters, you should gain about ½ to 1 pound a week.

Sugar Sense

If you're having trouble managing your blood sugar with self-injected insulin, your doctor may recommend an insulin pump for better control throughout the day. If your doctor doesn't suggest it and you're interested (go back and reread Chapter 9), you should bring it up.

This amount of weight increase is for women who start out with a normal weight. Your desirable body weight (DBW) before pregnancy really determines how much weight you should gain and how many calories you need. (Check back in Chapter 6 to reacquaint yourself with DBW.)

So here are the guidelines:

Pre-Pregnancy Weight	Total Weight Gain	Calories per Pound per Day*
Less than 90 percent DBW+	28-40 pounds	16-18
90-120 percent DBW	25-30 pounds	14
120-150 percent DBW	15-25 pounds	11
More than 150 percent DBW	Approx. 15 pounds	11

*Calories in second and third trimesters based on pre-pregnancy DBW; 300 total calories less in first trimester
+Unlikely in women with type 2 diabetes

The Rest of Your Pregnancy Diet

After eating, your glucose levels will primarily depend on the amount of carbohydrates you got in the meal. So the dietary challenge in pregnancy is to eat enough carbohydrates to avoid ketosis, but not so much that you wind up with post-meal high blood sugars.

Thus, the amount of carbohydrate in your diet is usually less than the amount you took in before pregnancy. For instance, you might aim for 40 percent of your daily calories instead of 50 to 55 percent.

Some doctors and dietitians like to spread the carbohydrates throughout the day. They suggest 10 percent at breakfast, 30 percent at lunch, 30 percent at supper, and the remaining 30 percent as snacks (including a bedtime snack).

Sugar Sense

Because your glucose rises more after breakfast than after other meals (because you generally have more insulin resistance at that time of day), a low-carbohydrate breakfast is a good idea.

This makes adjusting insulin doses a bit more complicated, however. So some providers prescribe three major meals and a bedtime snack, albeit with fewer carbohydrates at breakfast.

No matter which approach you choose, the goal is to keep your blood sugars at or close to normal. This reduces the need for insulin, and results in fewer too-large babies.

You'll also need to take supplemental iron (usually part of a good prenatal vitamin) and calcium, in addition to the prenatal vitamins your doctor will prescribe.

Exercising for Two

Pregnancy is no time to slack off on your physical activity. You just need to be smart about it. Most hospitals offer exercise programs specifically for pregnant women that combine some gentle stretching with moderate aerobic exercise. Swimming is an excellent activity when you're pregnant because the buoyancy of the water makes you feel lighter and you don't run the risk of becoming overheated.

And of course, you can always pull out your pedometer and keep walking. Just slow down as your belly gets larger, make sure your shoes are large enough (you may need bigger shoes as your pregnancy progresses), and walk on level, even ground—avoid any hikes in the woods for now.

Warning

Call your doctor immediately if you notice any of the following during your pregnancy:

- Ketones in your urine.
- Weight loss (your weight should be heading in the opposite direction, remember?)
- Sudden weight gain. Because you're seeing your healthcare team frequently, they should pick up on this. But if you notice a sudden increase in your weight from one day to the next, it could be a sign of pre-eclampsia.
- Glucose levels that are all over the map. Something's out of whack between your insulin, diet, and exercise. You need a tune-up.

When It's Time: Delivering the Baby

Back in the old days, women with diabetes who were close to their delivery date were hospitalized just to be on the safe side. Today, that no longer happens.

Nonetheless, in the week or two leading up to your due date, you can expect to undergo some extra testing to make sure the baby is doing okay. These may include an *ultrasound* to assess the baby's size, particularly if you plan to deliver vaginally, and fetal monitoring with either a *nonstress* or a *stress test* to make sure the baby is getting enough oxygen and his or her heart is functioning normally.

MedLingo _____

An **ultrasound** is a test that uses sound waves to create an image of the inside of your body. It is often used during pregnancy to assess the growth and development of the fetus. Another test used during pregnancy, primarily in late pregnancy, is a **non-stress test**. It involves strapping a fetal monitor around your belly to record the baby's heartbeat, providing a sense of the baby's health. During a **stress test**, the same measurements are recorded when the uterus is made to contract with medication.

Timing the Delivery

Your doctor will probably not want you to go past your due date; this just increases the risk that the baby will continue growing, making a vaginal delivery difficult. It also increases the risk of a stillbirth.

Thus, if you've reached your due date with no signs of labor, your doctor may decide to induce labor (depending on the severity of your diabetes, how well your blood glucose has been controlled throughout your pregnancy, and, of course, the condition of the baby). Your doctor may even decide to have you deliver the baby a couple of weeks early—just to be on the safe side.

Your doctor induces labor by breaking your water and having you walk around. If your contractions don't become regular within a few hours, you may be given labor-inducing drugs, such as pitocin, a synthetic form of the natural hormone oxytocin, which stimulates the uterus to contract.

You can probably plan on having a fairly medically intensive labor and delivery. This is no time to insist on "all natural," however. You are a high-risk pregnancy and your baby has a much higher risk of problems during delivery, including shoulder dystocia, in which the baby's shoulder gets wedged behind the mother's pubic bone. You can expect to have a fetal monitor, either internal or external, throughout labor to monitor the baby's heartbeat.

You'll also have your blood glucose levels measured frequently throughout labor, and probably receive intravenous insulin.

In some instances, your doctor may decide to simply schedule a planned cesarean section, determining that a vaginal delivery might be too risky to you and/or the baby.

After the Birth

Once the baby is born, don't worry if he or she has to be kept in a special nursery for a day or so. The doctors just want to monitor your infant's blood glucose levels, among other things, to make sure everything is okay.

As for you ... if you did not require insulin before pregnancy but had to take it during pregnancy, you probably won't need it now. If you were taking insulin before you became pregnant, the dose probably increased a lot during pregnancy. After delivery, you'll find that your need for insulin drops dramatically in the first few days, but then returns to its pre-pregnancy levels.

The Least You Need to Know

- ◆ Women with diabetes can become pregnant and successfully carry a healthy baby to term; it requires careful attention to blood glucose levels, however.

- ◆ Women with diabetes have a higher risk of having a miscarriage, stillbirth, or a baby born with birth defects; they are also more likely to encounter complications themselves, such as preeclampsia.

- ◆ Women with diabetes need to prepare for at least three months before getting pregnant.

- ◆ Pregnancy increases a woman's risk of retinopathy.

- ◆ Women with diabetes will usually be put on insulin during the pregnancy because pregnancy makes you more insulin resistant.

Chapter 15

On the Job

In This Chapter

◆ Diabetes and workplace discrimination

◆ The Americans with Diabetes Act

◆ Certain jobs that don't mix well with diabetes

◆ Tips for on-the-job health

You know by now that a diagnosis of diabetes means changes in every part of your life. Well, the workplace is no exception. Now in addition to deadlines, politics, and personalities, you've got to deal with glucose levels, hypoglycemia, and diet, along with absences for diabetes-related complications, doctor visits, and days when you're simply feeling too lousy to sit in a meeting or go on a sales call.

In this chapter, we show you how to cope with your diabetes on the job, how to make sure no one discriminates against you because you have diabetes, and how to tell your boss and co-workers about your condition—if you want to tell them.

We gratefully acknowledge the expert contributions to this chapter from Michael A. Greene, an attorney who specializes in employment discrimination. He is a past Chairman of the Board of Directors of the American

Diabetes Association (1993-1994) and has led the efforts to counter employment discrimination for people with diabetes. He has been the lead volunteer attorney for the American Diabetes Association in many of their groundbreaking cases. Mr. Greene is a partner in the law firm of Rosenthal & Greene, 1001 Southwest Fifth Avenue, Suite 1907, Portland, OR, 97204, (503) 228-3015.

Diabetes on the Job: Knowing Your Rights

Unlike some disabilities, like blindness, deafness, or mobility problems, your diabetes can remain a secret until you tell your employer about it. You're under no obligation to provide that information, however, and your employer is overstepping its bounds if anyone directly asks you.

Sometimes, keeping your diabetes to yourself is a smart move. For despite more than 15 years of progress since the passage of the American with Disabilities Act (ADA) in 1990, disability discrimination in the workplace is alive and well.

Although one survey (its findings are listed later in this section) found that just 1 percent of employers said they wouldn't hire someone with diabetes, other studies comparing people with diabetes to their nondiabetes siblings found that figure to be far higher. One study found that people with type 1 diabetes were more likely to be refused a job during their lifetime than their siblings. And not so surprisingly, those who told job interviewers about their diabetes were less likely to get the job than those who didn't.

People with diabetes were also less likely to be employed full time than their siblings, primarily because of disabilities related to their disease.

Our suggestion? Hold off on telling potential employers about your diabetes until the job is yours—just in case.

A survey of 2,500 business and industries in the United Kingdom in the late 1980s elicited some pretty interesting information about employers' attitudes toward employees with diabetes. Specifically …

- ◆ 1 percent claimed they would not consider someone with diabetes for a job.

- ◆ About a third didn't even know if they employed anyone with diabetes (see, it's easy to hide if you want to).

- ◆ More than one fourth of manufacturing employers said some of their jobs would be unsuitable for people with diabetes, including shift work, working at heights, strenuous work, etc.

♦ Firms that employed someone with diabetes said workers with diabetes had more sick days than nondiabetes employees.

♦ 16 percent of the firms employing people with diabetes said they didn't allow time off for doctor visits.

Although this study was carried out nearly 20 years ago in another country, later studies in this country find poorer employment possibilities for people with diabetes.

The American with Disabilities Act: What It Means for You

The good news is that once employed, studies today find little evidence of on-the-job discrimination against those with diabetes.

But just because large studies across wide populations show no on-the-job discrimination doesn't mean it doesn't exist. What you need to know is how to deal with it if you think it's happening to you.

The first tool in your toolbox against workplace discrimination is an understanding of the ADA (Americans with Disabilities Act). Passed in 1990, the Act represented a major milestone for people with all types of disabilities, guaranteeing them equal access in the workplace and public places. The goal of the act was to break down the barriers that prevent people with disabilities from fully participating in society. That means you.

Bet You Didn't Know

Unfortunately, your diabetes could put you out of the workplace with no help from discrimination. A 1994 study found that about 42 percent of those aged 18 to 69 with diabetes said they were unable to work, or were limited in the kind of work they could do, and about a third were so disabled they couldn't work at all. Overall, these high rates of disability translate into significant earning reductions for those with diabetes—more than $3,000 per year.

Yet another reason to keep a close eye on those glucose levels!

Here are the basic facts you should know about the ADA and diabetes:

♦ Generally, a potential or current employer cannot ask whether you have diabetes, or whether you use insulin or other prescription drugs.

◆ After you receive a job offer, however, an employer may ask about your health, including whether you have diabetes, and may require a medical examination (as long as it requires such examinations from *all* applicants).

◆ If your employer believes that your diabetes, or some other medical condition, may affect your ability to do your job, he or she can ask you about it and/or require a medical examination. However, this inquiry must be related to the specific requirements of the job and your capacity to carry them out.

◆ Your employer can also ask you about your diabetes if you have asked for a *reasonable accommodation* because of your diabetes, such as regular breaks to check your blood sugar, take medications, or get a snack, or if you're participating in a voluntary wellness program that focuses on the early detection, screening, and management of diseases such as diabetes.

◆ If you tell your employer that you have diabetes, the employer can only ask two questions: whether you need a reasonable accommodation and what type.

◆ Once you've been offered a job, your employer can't withdraw it just because you have diabetes as long as you're able to perform the "essential functions" of the job with or without *reasonable accommodations* and without posing a direct threat to safety.

◆ Your boss cannot tell your co-workers about your diabetes unless it's important that they know in order to do the job or meet your accommodations, or if you gave your permission.

MedLingo

The Equal Employment Opportunity Commission (EEOC) defines **reasonable accommodations** for people with diabetes to include such things as these:

◆ Breaks to eat or drink, take medication, or test your blood sugar levels.

◆ A private area to test blood sugar levels or take insulin.

◆ A place to rest until your blood sugar levels return to normal after a hypoglycemia episode.

◆ The ability to leave for treatment, recuperation, or training on managing diabetes.

◆ A modified work schedule or shift change.

◆ Allowing a person with diabetic neuropathy to use a stool.

Who's Covered

Unfortunately, the ADA has some limitations. It only applies to companies that employ 15 or more employees. While it applies to private companies, state and local governments, employment agencies, and labor unions, it does *not* apply to Native American tribes and tax-exempt private clubs. Neither does it apply to the federal government.

However, a similar law called the Federal Rehabilitation Act of 1973 provides ADA-like protection to federal employees, including federal contractors and organizations receiving federal funding.

If you work for a small company and are not covered by the ADA, check with your state EEOC office; most states have laws that fill in the gaps left by the ADA.

Warning

Your employer is not allowed to dismiss you because he or she fears your diabetes will affect health insurance premiums. Nor can your employer refuse to provide health insurance for you if it is provided for other employers who work a similar number of hours. Additionally, your employer cannot charge you a different premium for your health insurance than is charged to other employees.

Is Your Diabetes a Disability?

The EEOC says diabetes is considered a disability when it substantially limits one or more of your major life activites, such as eating or caring for yourself, or when it causes side effects or complications that could substantially limit these activities.

Even if your diabetes is not limiting your activities *now* because you're controlling it with lifestyle changes and medication, if it was limiting in the past (before it was treated or controlled) it might still be considered a disability.

Your diabetes is also considered a disability if it doesn't significantly affect your everyday activities but your employer treats you like it does, for instance, by assuming you're totally unable to work because you have diabetes.

Having said all that, if you do file a claim under the ADA, your case will be considered on its individual merits.

If You Suspect Discrimination

Here's what *not* to do if you think you've been discriminated against because of your diabetes: immediately file a claim with the EEOC. Instead, start with the action least likely to create a major ruckus.

The first step is to talk with your supervisor. Sometimes, what you perceive as discrimination might be a simple misunderstanding. If you aren't satisfied with the response from your supervisor, it's time to call in someone from human resources and/or your union.

Consider calling an attorney who specializes in the ADA. A simple letter or phone call might be all it takes to solve your problem.

Make sure you document every conversation about the alleged discrimination, including the incident itself.

If, after working through the company, you still aren't satisfied, now is the time to file a claim with the EEOC. You can find the number of your local office in your phone book's blue pages.

You generally have 180 days after the alleged discrimination occurred to file a claim. However, if your state has a contract arrangement with the EEOC to conduct the investigation, you may have up to 300 days. If the EEOC does not resolve the issue, you can always hire an attorney to file a lawsuit against the company.

Other on-the-Job Protections

If you work for a company with at least 50 employees who work at least 20 weeks a year, you also have some protection under the Family and Medical Leave Act (FMLA) if you need an extended period of time off for health reasons.

The FMLA provides up to 12 work weeks of unpaid leave during any 12-month period for one or more of the following reasons:

◆ The birth and care of the employee's newborn child

◆ Adoption or foster-care placement with the employee

◆ To care for an immediate family member (spouse, child, or parent) with a serious health condition

◆ To take medical leave when the employee is unable to work because of a serious health condition

To be eligible for the FMLA, you must have been employed by your employer for at least 12 months, and have been employed for at least 1,250 hours of service during the 12-month period immediately before the beginning of the leave.

Bet You Didn't Know

At one time in the not-so-distant past, employers and even governments forbade people who were taking insulin from certain jobs, such as driving a truck across state lines, flying an airplane, or serving on a police force.

The American Diabetes Association first tackled this issue in 1984, when it stated that "any person with diabetes, whether insulin dependent or noninsulin dependent, should be eligible for any employment for which he or she is otherwise qualified."

It took a lot of work and a lot of court cases, but the ADAs efforts have paid off. Today, it is illegal to have any blanket exclusions that prohibit people who take insulin from a particular job. Each case must be decided on its individual merits.

There is one exception. The military. Yup, that's right. If you take insulin to control your diabetes, you cannot serve in the military.

To Tell or Not to Tell

So now we come to the elephant in the living room. Should you tell your employer about your diabetes and, if you do, how do you do it?

The first thing to consider is that the ADA protects you from discrimination only if your employer knows you are disabled. It makes sense. How could you claim discrimination based on your diabetes if your boss didn't know you had diabetes?

Then you should consider the kind of job you do. If you operate heavy machinery, drive a vehicle, or work around dangerous equipment, and if you're prone to hypoglycemia, the two could be a dangerous match. In such instances, it's probably a good idea to talk to your boss about a reasonable accommodation, and if that's not practical, a possible reassignment.

Another good reason to tell your boss is to make sure that should something happen to you, like a hypoglycemic attack, your boss knows what's going on and how to handle it.

> **Sugar Sense**
>
> When you tell your boss about your diabetes, hand him or her a note from your doctor describing your condition, and your ability to work, along with any special needs you might have.

It's probably more important, however, to tell your co-workers because they'll be more likely to be around in case you need some help.

If you do decide to tell people at work about your disease, use the same basic techniques we described in Chapter 2 on telling your family and friends.

◆ Keep the information basic and simple.

◆ Keep explanations short and to the point.

◆ Simply tell them your condition, explain how you manage it, and assure them it will not interfere with your job.

◆ If you are taking insulin or a sulfonylurea agent, hypoglycemia is a potential problem. So it's a good idea to describe the signs of hypoglycemia to several people who work closest to you in case you need help.

Then get back to work!

Diabetes on the Job

Even though no one can discriminate against you for a particular job because you have diabetes, there are certain on-the-job situations that might interfere with good diabetes management. These include the following:

Sugar Sense

Why not use your diabetes as a selling point on the job? After all, it takes a lot personal strength and discipline to manage diabetes. You have to check your blood sugar, maintain a healthy weight, eat a prescribed diet at certain times, and manage a complex medication regimen. These are all evidence of your ability to handle complex tasks in the workforce with grace and competence.

◆ Shift work. Because you're getting up and going to bed at different times on different days, the change in schedule could throw off your diabetes management. If you take insulin, your doctor will need to work closely with you to find the best treatment schedule. Make sure your doctor knows when you eat, when you sleep, when you work, and whether you can eat and take insulin while working.

In this situation, you might want to consider an insulin pump, which affords more flexibility. Also make sure you get extra sleep; studies find that shift workers generally don't get enough sleep and we've already told you how that could affect your blood sugar levels.

- Physically intensive work. If you work in construction, unload containers, farm, or perform any of dozens of other physically intense work, you need to be aware of the effect of your job on your blood glucose. What you're doing is "exercising" all day long—and you'll need to take that into account in terms of what and when you eat, and how you use medications.

- Daily scheduling. If you take insulin or a sulfonylurea, you need to eat on time. If you're heading into a meeting that may delay your usual meal time, or aren't sure when it will end, make sure you eat something before the meeting or take a break to eat something during it.

On-the-Job Tips

There are certain things you can do to make handling your diabetes easier at work.

- Plan, plan, plan. For meals, glucose checks, insulin doses. Write it into your calendar, especially if you have automatic calendar systems that enable other people to schedule your appointments.

- Always carry something sweet or high carb with you, even if you're just going down the hall to the conference room. And keep snacks in your desk drawer or office fridge. If you don't have a desk, keep them in your pocket.

- Wear your MedicAlert bracelet at all times.

- Don't expect special favors in terms of sick days, lateness, etc. Your employer is under no obligation to give you more sick days than other employees, or to forgive your tardiness. If you miss too much work without permission, you could get fired.

The Least You Need to Know

- Diabetes doesn't have to interfere with your job—except in some circumstances.

- You may be protected under the Americans with Disability Act (ADA).

- It's up to you whether you tell your boss or co-workers about your condition.

- You cannot be excluded from a job just because you take insulin. Each case must be judged on an individual basis.

Part 4

Avoiding Complications

One of the worst things about diabetes is the risk of serious, life-threatening complications. In this section of the book, we tell you what they are and help you implement the kind of changes and lifestyle habits you need to avoid them. In Chapter 16, we cover your increased risk for heart disease, high blood pressure, and high cholesterol; in Chapter 17 we explain why diabetes is the leading cause of blindness in this country; and in Chapter 18 we help you maintain the health of your kidneys. Chapter 19 takes you through the numerous forms of nerve damage that can occur with diabetes, and in Chapter 20 you learn why taking care of your feet, mouth, and skin is so critical.

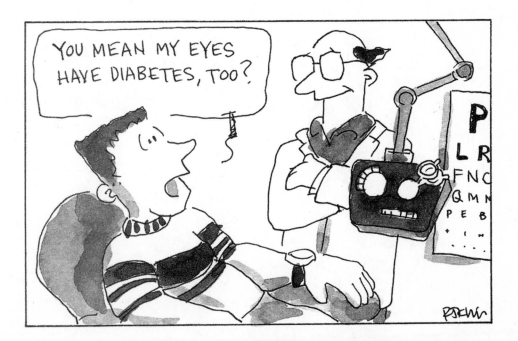

Chapter 16

Your Heart on Diabetes

In This Chapter

- Your risk for heart disease
- Types of heart disease
- High blood pressure and diabetes
- High cholesterol and diabetes
- Aspirin therapy for those with diabetes

Here's some news you may or may not want to hear. You probably won't die of diabetes. Nope. Instead, you're probably going to die of a heart attack, *stroke*, *heart failure*, or some other *cardiovascular disease*. Because as someone with diabetes, your risk of dying from cardiovascular disease—regardless of what type—is two to four times greater than someone without diabetes.

Plus, even though the overall rate of deaths from *heart disease* dropped significantly between 1970 and 1974, it dropped far less among those with diabetes.

In this chapter, we focus on why your risk of heart disease is so high and what you and your healthcare team can do about it.

Many Unaware of Higher Risks for Heart Disease

We know some of the answers as to why the risks are so much greater for people with diabetes and, more importantly, we know how to prevent many of those deaths. The problem is that neither people with diabetes nor their doctors are doing the things required to prevent or treat diabetic heart disease.

In fact, an American Diabetes Association survey found that 68 percent of those with diabetes were not aware of their increased risk for heart disease and stroke, and 60 percent didn't know they were at risk for high blood pressure and abnormal *lipids* (a fancy name for fats) in the blood, both of which increase their overall risk of heart disease and stroke.

> **Warning**
>
> Women with diabetes are less likely to be prescribed the three medications recommended to prevent heart disease in people with diabetes: an aspirin, a statin, and an *ACE inhibitor*.

> **MedLingo**
>
> **Cardiovascular disease (CVD)** refers to diseases of the arteries.
>
> **Heart disease** refers only to diseases of the heart, including CVD of the arteries within the heart and heart failure.
>
> A **stroke** occurs when an artery in the brain becomes blocked (ischemic stroke) or bursts (hemorrhagic stroke).
>
> **Lipids** refer to fats in the blood, primarily cholesterol and triglycerides.
>
> **Heart failure.** Heart failure means the heart muscle is too weak to pump blood throughout your body, as well as it should. It does NOT mean that the heart literally stops. Heart failure develops slowly over time and can have a large impact on a person's life and ability to perform daily activities of living, such as dressing, bathing, and getting around. You might also hear the phrase **congestive heart failure** used to describe heart failure; it refers to the backup of fluid in the lungs.
>
> An **ACE inhibitor** is a drug used to treat high blood pressure.

Starting with the Basics

First, let's start with the basics: Just what *is* heart disease and CVD, and what's the difference?

Heart disease refers only to diseases of the heart and the arteries within the heart. That would be things like heart attacks, heart failure, angina, and problems with your heartbeat, or electrical activity, the most common of which is atrial fibrillation.

Cardiovascular disease refers to diseases of the arteries within your entire body, including your brain and legs. So a stroke, for instance, would be a cardiovascular disease, not a heart disease. Similarly, problems with the arteries in the leg, called peripheral vascular disease, are another example of CVD that isn't heart disease.

Heart failure occurs when the heart gets too weak to pump out the blood normally and so fluid backs up into the lungs. CVD is one of the causes but there are other causes as well, such as high blood pressure, and microvascular changes in the small blood vessels of the heart. People with diabetes are more likely to develop heart failure than those who don't have diabetes.

Getting to Cardiovascular Specifics

Heart disease and cardiovascular disease are categories; underneath these categories are individual diseases and conditions that threaten your health. Because we talk about them throughout this chapter, it's important that you understand what they are and the differences among them:

- **Atherosclerosis** is thickening and hardening of the inside walls of the arteries. Basically, the inside of your arteries narrow as *plaque* and other gunk accumulate there. (This plaque is much different from the material that forms on your teeth, also called plaque.) The more plaque, the narrower the opening and the harder time blood has getting through.

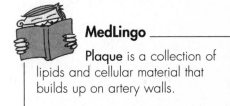

MedLingo

Plaque is a collection of lipids and cellular material that builds up on artery walls.

  Plus, the flow of blood itself could knock off some of that plaque. If a piece goes to the brain, it can cause a stroke. If the plaque comes from a larger artery within the heart and goes downstream to a smaller part of the artery, it can block blood flow and cause a heart attack.

- **Coronary heart disease (or coronary artery disease)** is the most common form of heart disease. It occurs when the coronary arteries become narrowed or clogged by cholesterol and other fat deposits, a major part of plaque, and can't supply enough blood to the heart.

◆ **Angina** is the pain or squeezing sensation you feel in your chest when your heart isn't getting enough blood. It's not a heart attack but it's a clear warning sign that one might be on the way. The most common reason for an angina attack is physical exertion; even something as simple as walking across the room could set off an attack in someone with bad heart disease.

◆ A **stroke** occurs when a blood clot blocks blood flow to the brain, or, less common, when a blood vessel in your brain bursts. Someone with diabetes has at least triple the risk of a stroke than someone without. If you're a woman with diabetes, your risk of stroke is greater than that of a man with diabetes.

◆ **High blood pressure (or hypertension).** Your blood pressure measures the force of the blood as it's pumped from your heart and travels through your blood vessels. Just as the force of water during a flood can damage the pipes and canals built to contain it, if your blood pressure is too high, it can damage the walls of your arteries. As mentioned above, up to three quarters of people with diabetes have high blood pressure and it's a risk factor for every type of CVD.

Diabetes and CVD: What's the Connection?

There are numerous reasons for the higher rates of CVD in people with diabetes. First, many of the risk factors for CVD—obesity, lack of physical exercise, hypertension, high triglyceride levels, and low HDL cholesterol levels—are present in people with type 2 diabetes.

Second, as you'll read throughout this section, one of the primary ways in which diabetes damages your body is by damaging blood vessels. The damage can occur in tiny blood vessels, like capillaries, in which case it's called *microvascular* disease and is generally a result of high blood sugar levels. Damage to these small blood vessels leads to the eye, kidney, and nerve complications of diabetes you'll read about later in this section and to the heart as described above.

Or, if the damage is to the big, blood-gushing arteries, it's called *macrovascular* disease. This latter form of blood vessel damage is to blame for your increased risk of CVD.

While managing your blood glucose levels is extremely important for preventing microvascular disease, low levels aren't going to have as much impact on your CVD risk. Instead, you have to take a multifaceted approach—losing weight, getting exercise, quitting smoking, reducing your blood pressure, and reducing your cholesterol and triglyceride levels—to make any significant difference in your risk of CVD.

Bet You Didn't Know

Although many women are more frightened of breast cancer than heart disease, they're much more likely to die of heart disease than breast cancer. In fact, heart disease is the number-one reason for death in women (and men) in the United States. Stroke is the third leading cause of death. So don't let your doctor ignore your risk factors for CVD and don't let anyone tell you that women don't have heart attacks. They do.

How Low Can You Go: Reducing Blood Pressure

Before we get too far into the blood pressure/diabetes link, let's talk about blood pressure itself. You've probably had your blood pressure taken dozens of times over your lifetime; but did you really understand the nurse when she gave the results?

It's not a difficult concept to understand. Blood pressure is measured in millimeters of mercury (mm Hg). You get two numbers, one on top of the other. The top number, called the systolic, measures the pressure when the *left ventricle* of your heart contracts; the bottom number, called the diastolic, measures the pressure when the ventricle relaxes.

MedLingo

The **left ventricle** is a heart chamber that pumps the blood out of the heart to the rest of the body through the arteries.

A blood pressure reading of 120/80 used to be considered great. But, like everything in life, even blood pressure guidelines are getting tougher.

Warning

When it comes to blood pressure, pay close attention to that top number. The systolic pressure is the one that seems to make the largest contribution to cardiovascular disease in those over 50. Reducing that figure seems to be the most effective way to reduce the kind of blood vessel damage from hypertension that can lead to kidney, heart, brain, or eye damage.

Nonetheless, the bottom, or diastolic figure, is also important. Anything over 120 mm Hg is an emergency; call your doctor immediately or head to the emergency room. Or if the top, or systolic, number is over 220 mm/Hg, do the same.

Today, if you have a blood pressure of 120/80 you're considered to have *prehypertension*. You need a blood pressure reading of *less* than 120/80 to be considered normal. Some studies suggest that the optimum blood pressure should be 115/75—a big difference from the old goal.

MedLingo

End stage renal disease refers to the point at which your kidneys can no longer clean out your blood, and you must go on **dialysis** three days a week to take over your kidney function.

A large body of evidence finds that controlling blood pressure levels in people with diabetes to less than 130/80 (yeah, another thing to control, more numbers to memorize) will significantly reduce your risk of CVD and stroke, as well as the development of kidney disease, which often leads to *end stage renal disease (ESRD)*.

So let's recap: Controlling your blood pressure could keep you from having a heart attack or stroke, having to go on *dialysis*, or going blind. Sounds like a good investment to us!

Sugar Sense

Unfortunately, studies find about one third of people with diabetes diagnosed with hypertension didn't know about the diagnosis, and almost half of those with high blood pressure were untreated!

So the first step in controlling hypertension is getting your blood pressure checked every time you go to the doctor. You should also check it a couple times a month yourself, either at the drugstore or with a home blood pressure monitor.

Getting the Numbers Down

If you have diabetes and hypertension, your doctor should try to get your blood pressure down below 130/80 mm Hg. Initially, you can try lifestyle changes, but if they don't work, and they often don't, you'll also need medication.

You'll likely be able to give it a go with just lifestyle changes—diet, exercise, stress reduction—if your starting blood pressure is between 120/80 and 139/89. In this instance, if you're already working to eat a healthy diet, lose weight, and get regular physical activity, about the only thing we'd add on the lifestyle end has to do with your salt intake.

Although it affects some people worse than others, salt, or sodium, is most likely a primary contributor to hypertension. A 1999 study published in the *Journal of the American Medical Association* found an increased risk of stroke in overweight people who ate a lot of salt in their diets.

Those people were in trouble in other ways, too. They were 89 percent more likely to die from stroke, 44 percent more likely to die from coronary heart disease, 61 percent more likely to die from all cardiovascular disease, and 39 percent more likely to die from all causes than those who got just 2,300 mg or less of sodium a day.

However, if the people in this study weren't overweight, then they had no higher risk of dying, regardless of how much salt they ate. So, if you want to eat more salt, better lose that extra weight first.

Still, regardless of weight, the typical American diet, with 3,600 to 4,000 mg of sodium a day, is simply too high in salt. And you don't need it. Because salt is an acquired taste, meaning you like it because you're used to it, if you gradually started to cut back a little at a time you'd find in a few weeks that you don't need as much of it to flavor foods.

The easiest way to cut back? Cut out processed foods. Processed foods are powerhouses of sodium, added to improve shelf life, color, texture, and flavor.

So instead of buying canned chicken soup, make up a huge pot on the weekend and freeze in individual servings. Forget packaged dinners in favor of fresh. Avoid canned tomatoes, canned beans, and other canned veggies and buy frozen or fresh. Even packaged sweets have surprisingly high levels of sodium.

Sugar Sense _____

Like sugar, the language of salt and sodium can be tricky. So when you're reading labels, don't be fooled by the phrases of food manufacturers. Here's what they really mean—according to the U.S. Food and Drug Administration (FDA).

- Sodium free or salt free: Less than 5 mg per serving
- Very low sodium: 35 mg or less per serving
- Low sodium: 140 mg or less of sodium
- Low sodium meal: 140 mg or less of sodium per 3.5 ounces
- Reduced or less sodium: At least 25 percent less sodium than the regular version
- Light in sodium: 50 percent less sodium than the regular version
- Unsalted or no salt added: No salt added to the product during processing

Drugs to Drop Blood Pressure

If your blood pressure is 130/80 mm Hg or higher after trying lifestyle modifications, your doctor should probably start you on one or more blood pressure medications. In fact, don't be surprised if you eventually need three or more! The drug(s) that your doctor prescribes will depend on numerous factors, including complications you may have in addition to hypertension. For instance, beta blockers may make peripheral vascular disease worse although they might be the preferred choice in someone who has had a heart attack. Certain diuretics don't work well if kidney function is too low. Other medications shouldn't be used if the potassium levels in the blood are too high.

The main classes of drugs to treat hypertension are these:

◆ *Angiotensin-converting enzyme (ACE) inhibitors.* By interfering with your body's production of *angiotensin*, a chemical that makes arteries contract, ACE inhibitors relax blood vessels. Studies find these drugs to be beneficial in reducing rates of heart attack, stroke, and angina, and preventing the progression of kidney disease.

MedLingo

Angiotensin is a chemical that makes arteries contract, or shrink, restricting blood flow which increases blood pressure.

◆ *Angiotensin II receptor blockers (ARBs).* These drugs do just what their name says: They prevent angiotensin from getting into cells to do their job. They also seem to have some benefit in preventing the progression of kidney disease. Because of the beneficial effects on the kidney, either an ACE inhibitor or an ARB should be the first drug used to treat hypertension (unless there is a some reason you shouldn't take it).

◆ *Diuretics.* These drugs work in the kidney and flush excess water and sodium from the body. If kidney function is normal, they should be the second drug added in people with diabetes if an ACE inhibitor or an ARB aren't doing the job.

◆ *Calcium channel blockers.* These drugs treat hypertension by helping relax blood vessels. Some also reduce your heart rate.

◆ *Beta blockers.* These drugs partially block one kind of nerve signal to your blood vessels and your heart. This relaxes your blood vessels and lowers your heart rate as well as the amount of blood your heart releases to the rest of your body.

◆ *Alpha-blockers.* These drugs partially block another kind of nerve signal to blood vessels. This, in turn, enables blood to pass more easily through the blood vessels resulting in lower blood pressure.

◆ *Alpha beta-blockers.* These drugs block both kinds of nerve signals to the blood vessels (alpha and beta).

◆ *Nervous system* inhibitors, also called sympathetic nerve inhibitors. These drugs relax blood vessels by controlling nerve signals that cause blood vessels to constrict. Thus, they widen blood vessels, enabling blood to flow more easily and reducing blood pressure.

◆ *Vasodilators.* These drugs work as a kind of muscle relaxer for muscles in blood vessel walls, enabling the vessels to open wider, thus reducing pressure.

MedLingo

There are several classes of blood pressure medications. **Angiotensin-converting enzyme (ACE) inhibitors** interfere with the production of *angiotensin*, a chemical that makes arteries contract, to relax blood vessels. **Angiotensin II receptor blockers (ARBs)** prevent angiotensin from getting into cells to do their job. **Diuretics** flush excess water and sodium from the body. **Calcium channel blockers** help relax blood vessels. **Alpha and beta blockers (and alpha/beta blockers)** partially block nerve signals to blood vessels and the heart to relax vessels and lower heart rate. **Nervous system inhibitors**, also called **sympathetic nerve inhibitors**, relax blood vessels by controlling nerve signals that cause blood vessels to constrict. **Vasodilators** work as a kind of muscle relaxer for muscles in blood vessel walls, enabling the vessels to open wider.

Of Cholesterol and Other Blood Lipids

We've talked some throughout this book about the effect of diabetes on cholesterol, both good and bad. You already know that people with type 2 diabetes are more likely to have low levels of HDL (good) cholesterol and high levels of triglycerides, another type of blood fat.

Even more worrisome, although LDL (bad) cholesterol levels aren't usually increased in people with diabetes, they are more likely to be carried around the bloodstream as small, dense LDL cholesterol particles. These particles are more likely to become oxidized and cause changes to the walls of your arteries, resulting in the formation of plaque.

As you know, high levels of small, dense LDL cholesterol particles and triglycerides, combined with low levels of HDL cholesterol, significantly increase your risk of cardiovascular disease. The good news is that we're getting very, very good at treating these risk factors, with some excellent medications that can literally save your life.

Insulin Resistance at Work Again

So just why do people with type 2 diabetes have this increased risk for abnormal levels of blood lipids? Blame that ole' insulin resistance.

Although the evidence is still forthcoming, we're pretty sure that insulin resistance underlies the mechanism at work here. The theory is that the high levels of insulin seen in people with insulin resistance increase the liver's production of a form of lipids known as *very low-density lipoprotein (VLDL)*. These particles carry a lot of triglycerides.

These VLDLs seem to result in the increased production of those smaller, denser LDL particles we talked about earlier. In turn, the increased levels of triglycerides trigger a chemical process leading to reduced HDL cholesterol levels. Think of it as a series of connected circles, with one change in blood lipids resulting in another change resulting in another change, and so on and so on.

And that's just the tip of the metabolic iceberg!

So What's It All Mean?

Why care about all these numbers? Simple. Studies find that an increase of just 89 mg/dl in triglyceride levels increases coronary risk significantly, 14 percent for men and 37 percent for women. As described above, small, dense LDL particles cause changes on the arterial walls that result in CVD. On the other hand, low HDL cholesterol levels also increase the risk of heart disease.

Cholesterol by the Numbers

In general, ideal cholesterol levels depend on many things, including one's family history, age, weight, whether you smoke, have kidney disease, or whether you have a previous history of heart disease. Depending on how many of these risk factors you have, any LDL level above 100 mg/dL might be considered too high. However, in people with diabetes, the CVD risk is so high that the ideal LDL cholesterol level should be less than 100 mg/dL. And if you already have CVD, levels below 70 mg/dL are recommended.

Nonetheless, there are some general guidelines for healthy people without diabetes who have few or none of these risk factors.

LDL Cholesterol Level	Category
Less than 100 mg/dL	Optimal
100-129 mg/dL	Near optimal
130-159 mg/dL	Borderline high
160-189 mg/dL	High
190 mg/dL and above	Very high

Your LDL cholesterol levels are just one part of the equation. You also want to know your HDL cholesterol levels. Here, you want your HDL cholesterol levels to be high—the higher the better. Overall, here's how HDL cholesterol shakes out:

HDL Cholesterol Level	Category
Less than 40 mg/dL	Risky
40-59 mg/dL	Average
60 mg/dL and above	Protective

Unfortunately, you are not considered healthy; you already have one major risk factor for heart disease: diabetes.

Thus, ideal blood lipid levels for you are an LDL cholesterol less than 100 mg/dL, a triglyceride level less than 150 mg/dL, and an HDL greater than 40 mg/dL for men and more than 50 mg/dL for women.

Getting to Goal

Of course, lifestyle changes are usually the first thing recommended for most people with abnormal lipid levels. You, however, are not most people. It's highly unlikely you're going to be able to manage your cholesterol levels with diet and exercise alone.

In fact, these days, some physicians recommend that everyone with diabetes be started on a *statin* regardless of their cholesterol levels. The reason?

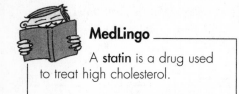

MedLingo

A **statin** is a drug used to treat high cholesterol.

The 2003 publication of the landmark Heart Protection Study in the journal *Lancet*. The study found that using 40 mg daily of one of the statins, Zocor (simvastatin), cut the risk of cardiovascular problems in people with diabetes by about a third, even in those whose cholesterol levels were normal.

Another report in the same journal in the summer of 2004, called the CARD Study, found the same thing. Ten milligrams of Lipitor (atorvastatin), another statin, reduced CVD by 48 percent in diabetic patients with LDL cholesterol concentrations slightly above or even less than 100 mg/dl.

Overall, study researchers from the Heart Protection Study said using a statin to reach goal LDL cholesterol levels could prevent 45 out of every 1,000 people with diabetes from suffering at least one major cardiovascular problem, such as angina or a heart attack. Researchers from the CARD study said it could prevent at least 37 major vascular events per 1,000 people treated for four years.

Unfortunately, raising HDL cholesterol levels is not as easy as reducing LDL cholesterol levels. Two of the drugs described above will increase HDL cholesterol levels only a little bit. The best way to do it is with an intensive exercise program, which is very helpful for other things as well, such as insulin resistance, weight loss, and hypertension.

Sugar Sense

The American Diabetes Association has come up with a clever way to help you remember what you need to do to reduce your overall risk of heart disease. They call it the ABCs of diabetes:

◆ An A1C (glycated hemoglobin) result less than 7 percent

◆ A blood pressure reading less than 130/80 mm Hg

◆ An LDL cholesterol reading of less than 100 mg/dl

The last two have been found to significantly reduce the risk of heart disease, and the first is very beneficial for protecting the eye, kidney, and nerves from complications so common in those with diabetes.

Sussing Out the Statins

In addition to Zocor and Lipitor, five other statins are approved for marketing in the United States: Lescol (fluvastatin), Mevacor (lovastatin), Pravachol (pravastatin), and Crestor (rosuvastatin), and the extended release form of Mevacor, Altocor.

Statins, also called HMG-CoA reductase inhibitors, work by partially blocking the enzyme HMG-CoA, hence their name. This enzyme controls how quickly your body produces cholesterol. Statins also increase your body's ability to get rid of LDL cholesterol, and even show some benefits in terms of reducing triglycerides and increasing HDL cholesterol levels, albeit relatively small benefits.

The most common side effects from statins include gastrointestinal problems, like nausea or stomach upset. Much less common side effects include liver or kidney damage, muscle pain or weakness, and a very rare condition called *rhabdomyolysis*, the breakdown of muscle tissue.

Your doctor may check your liver enzymes and other chemicals markers for the first few months to make sure you're not experiencing any of these problems.

> **CAUTION**
>
> **Warning**
>
> Let your doctor know immediately if you experience any significant muscle pain, weakness, tenderness, lethargy, fever, dark urine, nausea, or vomiting—all possible signs of rhabdomyolysis. Rhabdomyolysis is a very rare condition that results in the breakdown of muscle tissue. It is sometimes associated with statin use.

Beyond Statins

Statins are not the only tool in the cholesterol-lowering toolbox. Your doctor has several other medications from which to choose, including the following:

♦ **Bile acid resins.** Three primary bile acid resins are prescribed in the United States. They bind the cholesterol produced by the liver and help eliminate it in the stool. They typically lower cholesterol levels by 10 to 20 percent and are added to a statin if the LDL cholesterol goal of less than 100 mg/dl is not met. They are taken with each meal and can cause bloating, abdominal cramps, and diarrhea. Bile acid resins may also *raise* triglycerides, however, so if your triglyceride levels are already high, it's unlikely you'd be prescribed this drug.

♦ **Niacin.** This compound is more commonly known as nicotinic acid, a water-soluble B vitamin, but the over-the-counter version won't do it for you. You need a prescription formula. Taken before meals, it lowers both cholesterol and triglyceride levels and raises HDL cholesterol levels.

However, it has some temporary unpleasant side effects (itching, tingling, feeling hot). These side effects are less common with an extended release form. Taking an aspirin 30 minutes before the niacin also minimizes side effects. Finally, high doses of niacin can cause liver trouble as well as raise blood sugars.

♦ **Fibrates.** These drugs reduce triglycerides by 20 to 50 percent and usually raise HDL cholesterol 10 to 15 percent. However, they have little effect on LDL cholesterol levels.

♦ **Cholesterol absorption inhibitors.** This new class of drugs lowers cholesterol by preventing it from being absorbed in the intestine. The first approved drug in this class is Zetia (ezetimibe). Studies find that it lowers LDL cholesterol about 20 percent. Since it has few side effects, it is more likely to be added to a statin than a bile acid resin if the statin does not lower LDL cholesterol levels to less than 100 mg/dl.

Take One Aspirin and Call Me in the Morning

Ah, the lowly aspirin. It sits in every medicine cabinet in nearly every house in the country, rattles around purses and briefcases, and hides out in desk drawers. But did you know that aspirin may very well be one of the most powerful drugs around when it comes to reducing your risk of heart attack and stroke, and helping you live through a heart attack?

It's so helpful, in fact, that the American Diabetes Association recommends that people with diabetes over the age of 40 take a daily low-dose aspirin to help prevent a heart attack. Anyone who has had a heart attack, whether they have diabetes or not, should be taking an aspirin unless there is some reason (such as allergies or stomach problems) not to.

Aspirin seems to have numerous effects on the heart. Most important, it makes blood cells more slippery and less likely to clot. It also soothes inflammation in the arteries, which helps protect clumps of plaque or blood clots from breaking off and causing trouble.

It doesn't take much aspirin to benefit: Studies find that between 75 and 100 milligrams is enough to reduce the risk of heart attack or angina. This is known as "low-dose aspirin therapy," and most aspirin brands come in low-dose formulations of 81 mg.

Aspirin is not totally benign, however. It can cause stomach problems in some people. Because it acts on the overall system that affects bleeding, aspirin also occasionally increases the risk of bleeding from the stomach, kidneys, and colon, and it may rarely increase the risk of a form of stroke caused not by a blood clot, but by bleeding in the brain.

Because heart attacks are so common in people with diabetes and the effect of aspirin is so beneficial in reducing this risk, the risk, however, of these occasional side effects should not stop you from taking a low-dose aspirin.

But check with your doctor before you start.

CAUTION

Warning _____

Women with diabetes are much less likely to be on aspirin therapy than men. Overall, between 1988 and 1994, only 20 percent of all those with diabetes—women and men—took aspirin regularly, leading government researchers to conclude that "major efforts are needed to increase aspirin use among those with diabetes." This has had some effect, because in 2001, studies found that half of those with diabetes over the age of 35 were taking aspirin. Again, however, significantly fewer women than men were taking it. And that still leaves an awful lot of people who should be taking aspirin, but aren't.

The Least You Need to Know

- Since you have diabetes, your risk of cardiovascular disease and stroke is much higher than someone without diabetes.

- You are much more likely to have high blood pressure, high triglyceride and low HDL cholesterol levels, as well as small, dense LDL cholesterol particles, all of which significantly increase your risk of heart disease.

- You should aim for a blood pressure of less than 130/80 mm Hg.

- You should aim for an LDL level of less than 100 mg/dl, an HDL level over 40 (if you're male) and over 50 (if you're female), and a triglyceride level less than 150 mg/dl.

- You are likely to be put on medications for both high blood pressure and abnormal blood lipids.

- As someone with diabetes over the age of 40, you should probably be taking a low-dose aspirin every day to reduce your risk of heart attack.

Take Good Care of Your Eyes

In This Chapter

- Diabetic retinopathy: a common and feared problem
- Types and progression of diabetic retinopathy
- Prevention of diabetic retinopathy
- Treating diabetic retinopathy
- Other eye conditions

Back in the very old days, few people ever went blind from diabetes. That's because very few people with diabetes ever lived long enough for the complication to develop. Today, however, diabetic retinopathy is one of the most dreaded complications of diabetes and the leading cause of blindness in adults under 65.

An estimated 5.5 million adults with diabetes—both types—have diabetic retinopathy, and another 10,000 are diagnosed with the condition every year.

Although it is much more common in people with type 1 diabetes (nearly all will have some level of retinopathy within 20 years of their diagnosis), one fourth of those with type 2 diabetes will have retinopathy within two years of their diagnosis, and 60 percent will have some form of the disease 20 or more years after diagnosis.

Plus, people with diabetes are more likely to develop other eye-related conditions that could steal their sight, including *glaucoma* and *cataracts*.

The good news? If your retinopathy is detected and treated early, there's no reason in the world why you have to lose your sight. This chapter tells you all you need to know.

MedLingo

Glaucoma is a condition in which fluid doesn't drain normally from the eye. The build-up of fluid increases pressure in the eye, eventually destroying the **optic nerve,** the bundle of nerves that travels from the *retina* to the brain. The **retina** is the light-sensitive membrane covering the back wall of the eyeball that connects the images coming into the eye with the optic nerve.

Cataracts are cloudy lenses of the eye, generally age related.

R is for Retinopathy

Basically, diabetic retinopathy is a microvascular disease, affecting the tiny blood vessels in the back of your eyes. When the blood sugar remains high over many years, the walls of the blood vessels weaken and some blood and fluid leak out.

Bet You Didn't Know
The American Diabetes Association estimates that up to 21 percent of people with type 2 diabetes already have retinopathy, while the UK Prospective Diabetes Study (UKPDS) study found that 34 percent had retinopathy when first diagnosed. That could be because studies find that retinopathy begins to develop an average of five years before type 2 diabetes is even diagnosed. So by the time you know you've got something to worry about, you could be halfway to losing your sight!

Eventually the blood vessels get blocked, and new, weaker ones form to get around the blockage. These new vessels can break, sending even more blood into the eye and creating quite a mess, as you'll read.

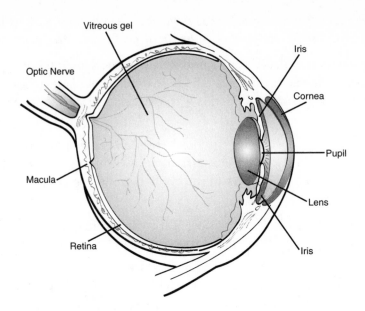

The Human Eye ©National Eye Institute

Three Types of Retinopathy

There are three main types of diabetic retinopathy.

The first type is *nonproliferative diabetic retinopathy (NPDR)*. This type, also called *background retinopathy*, represents the early stage of retinopathy. In this type of retinopathy, three things happen:

- The walls of the blood vessels weaken and bulge out forming small sacs. These are called *microaneurysms*.

- The liquid part of the blood leaks out, causing *exudates* on the retina.

- The blood cells themselves leak out causing *hemorrhages* on the retina.

This sounds bad, but it usually doesn't cause any problems with vision unless *macular edema* occurs.

Macular edema is really part of NPDR, but it's considered a second type of diabetic retinopathy because it can cause loss of vision. The *macula* is the part of the eye in which vision is sharpest. If fluid from blood vessels leak here, the macula swells and vision becomes blurred. Macular edema is especially common in older people with diabetes.

The third type of diabetic retinopathy is called *proliferative diabetic retinopathy (PDR)*. It gets its name from the new blood vessels that grow, or proliferate, on the retina.

This type of retinopathy occurs as NPDR gets worse, the blood vessels become blocked, and the retina is starved for oxygen. The retina sends out distress signals and new blood vessels grow to supply the retina with oxygen, a process called *neovascularization*.

These vessels, however, are weak and prone to break, resulting in leaking blood. This leaking blood often leaves the back of the eye, making its way into the *vitreous*, the clear, gel-like substance that fills the center of the eye between the lens and the retina.

Blood in the vitreous can really block your vision. If it clears (which can take weeks to months), your vision returns. Sometimes this doesn't clear, and you're left with some loss of vision.

A vitreous hemorrhage can also lead to another big problem. As the blood clots, it shrinks. But since part of the blood is attached to the retina, it can pull the retina off the back of the eye, kind of like a scab pulling your skin together, causing a *detached retina*.

This definitely causes loss of vision. (Fortunately, if diagnosed early enough, *ophthalmologists* can often tack the retina back, restoring your vision.)

Sometimes new blood vessels grow on the *iris*, the colored part of your eye, blocking the flow of fluid from the eye. This leads to a build-up of fluid, or increased pressure, resulting in a condition called *neovascular glaucoma*, which is very painful and will eventually damage the optic nerve and lead to blindness.

MedLingo

In nonproliferative diabetic retinopathy (NPDR), also called **background retinopathy,** the blood vessels first weaken bulge, causing **microaneurysms,** or tiny tears. Then the blood vessels get so weak that the fluid part of the blood leaks out, forming deposits on the retina called **exudates.** When the red blood cells leak out, one can see small **hemorrhages** on the retina.

If fluid from leaking blood vessels results in swelling of the macula, the small spot in the retina where vision is sharpest, it is called **macular edema.** Exudates here can interfere with vision.

An Ounce of Prevention

The best way to prevent diabetic retinopathy is by maintaining blood sugars (as reflected in your A1C test) near normal.

If you do develop retinopathy, the best way to prevent blindness is with early diagnosis and treatment—before you even have any symptoms. That requires regular eye exams with either an ophthalmologist or an *optometrist* who has a lot of experience looking at retinas.

To get the best look at your retina, your eyes should be dilated. In fact, if you combine yearly dilated eye screenings with early laser treatment if retinopathy is found (more about that later), it is very unlikely that you will go blind.

As to which doctor is best, well, given your diabetes, you're better off with an ophthalmologist who specializes in diabetes. Frankly, most non-ophthalmologists are not very good at diagnosing retinopathy (especially since they are unlikely to dilate the eyes because it takes a lot of time).

If your regular ophthalmologist finds evidence of retinopathy, an ophthalmologist who specializes in diseases of the retina, called a retinal specialist, will likely see you. He or she may want to see you about every six months.

> **CAUTION**
>
> **Warning**
>
> Make sure you have someone else drive you home from your eye doctor exams. Your eyes remain dilated for many hours after the exam, making clear vision difficult. You should also wear sunglasses because your eyes will be sensitive to light.

The Screening Exam

During a screening exam, the doctor should test your vision to see how well you're seeing. He or she will then dilate your pupils with special drops, and use an *ophthalmoscope* to examine the back of your eye for any blood vessel changes after dilating the pupils. This is called *funduscopy* or a funduscopic examination.

If you do have diabetic retinopathy, the retina specialist may want a more detailed look at your blood vessels via *fluorescein angiography*. This involves a special digital camera that takes pictures of your eye and analyzes the blood circulation around the retina. After a few pictures, a special dye (*fluorescein*) is injected into your arm, where it travels through your blood vessels, including those in your eye.

The doctor then takes additional photographs as the dye travels through your eye to get a detailed look at how diabetes has affected your retinal blood vessels. These photographs are saved and compared to new pictures taken during subsequent eye exams.

The ophthalmologist will also check the pressure in your eye to see if you have glaucoma. To do this, the doctor places a special dye in your eye (don't worry, it only stings a bit) and takes some measurements.

MedLingo

An **optometrist** primarily performs routine eye exams and fittings for glasses and contact lenses.

During these routine eye exams, the doctor may conduct an examination called **funduscopy**, using a special instrument called an **ophthalmoscope** to examine your retina.

Another test, called a **fluorescein angiography,** involves injecting dye (**fluorescein**) into your arm so that it travels to the eye, enabling the doctor to better visualize any blood vessel problems and photograph them with a special camera.

Treating Diabetic Retinopathy

Once early diabetic retinopathy is diagnosed, your doctor will want to begin treatment as soon as possible to prevent the retinopathy from getting worse. The first step is making sure you're managing your blood sugars well. In fact, the best way to slow the progression of early diabetic retinopathy is with strict blood sugar control. Otherwise, your retinopathy will only get worse, regardless of treatment.

The second step is controlling high blood pressure. High blood pressure, or hypertension, significantly increases the risk of diabetic retinopathy. And, like diabetic retinopathy itself, hypertension is often silent, with no symptoms until the disease has gotten really serious. So reread Chapter 16 and make sure your regular doctor checks you closely for hypertension and does whatever it takes—medication and otherwise—to get your pressure under control.

The third step, and a very important one, is to stop smoking. High blood sugars, high blood pressure, and smoking are three risk factors associated with diabetic retinopathy.

There's really no medication available yet for diabetic retinopathy. Thus, laser surgery is the preferred treatment for more advanced retinopathy, including macular edema. Surgery won't reverse retinopathy, but it can contain it, hopefully preventing it from getting worse and damaging your vision more.

Bet You Didn't Know

Diabetic retinopathy and diabetic nephropathy, or kidney disease, which you read more about in Chapter 18, tend to hang together. So if you have one, you're much more likely to have the other. Another potential risk factor is high blood cholesterol. It turns out that high cholesterol is associated with more exudates; lowering cholesterol reduces exudates (although this doesn't actually affect your vision). So make sure that if you have one of these three conditions, you and your doctor are on the lookout for the others.

Laser Surgery

All laser surgeries are performed in the doctor's office or an outpatient clinic. The doctor dilates your pupil as discussed previously, and uses drops to numb your eye. You may see flashes of bright green or red light during the procedure, which may make your eyes sting.

After the surgery, you're free to go. Make sure you have someone drive you home. Your doctor may give you some drops to prevent any post-surgical discomfort.

Two side effects of laser treatment are loss of *peripheral vision* (side vision) and greater difficulty seeing at night.

Laser surgery is usually not a one-time procedure. Each episode may require several visits because the doctor makes hundreds of laser burns in the retina, especially during panretinal photocoagulation. Also, once you've had laser treatment, you may need it again several times during your lifetime.

MedLingo

Peripheral vision is the ability to see objects and movement outside of the direct line of vision.

> **Sugar Sense** _____
>
> Under the American Academy of Ophthalmology's EyeCare America initiative, Medicare beneficiaries age 65 and older who have diabetes and haven't had a medical eye exam in the past three years can be matched with a volunteer ophthalmologist in their area. You'll receive a comprehensive eye exam and up to one year of follow-up care at no out-of-pocket cost for any disease diagnosed at the initial exam. To see if you are eligible for a referral to a nearby EyeCare America volunteer ophthalmologist, call toll-free 1-800-272-EYES (3937) or visit EyeCare America.

Focal Surgery

In one form of laser surgery, called *focal laser*, also called *photocoagulation*, the doctor aims a laser, a high-energy beam of light, at the blood vessels leaking blood, sealing them up so that they stop leaking.

The laser may also be used to destroy parts of the retina that no longer work because of a stopped-up blood supply. This prevents those areas from sending out signals that result in the growth of new blood vessels, leading to PDR.

Focal laser is also used to treat macular edema. Although it won't improve your vision, it will stabilize it so that it doesn't get any worse. That's why it's so important to have yearly dilated eye exams to pick up this condition before much vision loss occurs.

Hundreds of Laser Burns

If you have proliferative retinopathy, the doctor will use a *scatter laser treatment*, also called *panretinal photocoagulation*. During this procedure, the doctor makes hundreds of small laser burns.

> **MedLingo** _____
>
> **Focal laser** is a treatment for proliferative diabetic retinopathy in which a laser is used to seal leaking blood vessels.
>
> **Scatter laser treatment**, also called **panretinal photocoagulation**, uses a laser to destroy many different areas in the retina to prevent the signals that lead to new blood vessel growth.

We're not quite sure why this treatment works, but researchers suspect that it may thin the retina, increasing the amount of oxygen that can get to it, or induce parts of the eye to produce certain chemicals that prevent the growth of new blood vessels. It is also used to shrink and destroy existing abnormal blood vessels.

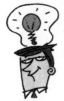

Sugar Sense

Whether you're having problems with your vision because of your diabetes or simply because you're getting older, the following tips will help:

♦ Increase the font size on the computer. You can also increase the size of the displayed document. For instance, you can view it at 125 percent of its original size.

♦ For better driving at night, turn on the map light in your car. Just that little illumination will make your pupils contract, reducing the amount of peripheral light that enters your eyes and enabling you to see farther.

♦ Carry eye drops. As you age, your eyes dry out. Some eye conditions may also cause this condition. Liquid tears and other eye drops can keep your eyes moist and feeling more comfortable.

♦ Use high-wattage bulbs in your lamps. The days of getting by on 40-watt bulbs are over.

Vitrectomy: Serious Surgery

If you have a lot of blood in the vitreous of your eye, as discussed above, you may require a *vitrectomy* to clear your vision. In this procedure, you are given either a local or general anesthetic and may stay overnight in the hospital.

During a vitrectomy, the doctor cuts a tiny incision in your eye and then removes the bloodied vitreous gel, replacing it with a salt solution. This is possible because the vitreous gel is mostly water anyway. At the same time, the doctor will repair your retina if it's detached, and remove any abnormal blood vessels that caused the original bleeding.

Sugar Sense

A new approach under investigation in people with macular edema whose vision continues to get worse despite laser treatment is the injection of *corticosteroids*, anti-inflammatory drugs, in the back of the eye. Some small studies find that this can improve vision. A larger, controlled study is now underway to see if this new treatment really works.

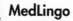
MedLingo

Corticosteroids are anti-inflammatory drugs injected into the back of the eye to treat macular edema.

After you go home, your eyes may be red and sensitive for a few days. You'll have to wear an eye patch to protect your eye for a few days or weeks, and use antibiotic drops to prevent infection.

If you need the procedure done on both eyes, your doctor will schedule the second eye after the first one heals.

Other Eye Conditions

As noted earlier, in addition to diabetic retinopathy, people with diabetes are also more likely to develop other eye conditions than people without diabetes. These include the following:

♦ **Glaucoma.** Glaucoma is a condition in which fluid from the eye doesn't flow normally through the proper channels, but instead builds up behind the eye. This, in turn, increases the pressure in the eye, eventually destroying the optic nerve.

As discussed earlier, people with diabetes are prone to a rare form called neovascular glaucoma. But they're also twice as likely as someone without diabetes to develop run-of-the-mill glaucoma. There are several treatments for glaucoma, including medications, laser surgery, and other forms of surgery.

Warning

See your eye doctor immediately if you notice flashing lights (especially only in one eye) or any sudden change in your vision, such as a sudden increase in floaters you can see. This could be a sign of a major problem, such as bleeding.

♦ **Cataracts.** Cataracts form when the lens of the eye clouds over, interfering with sight. Although cataracts typically develop in people over the age of 65, they occur earlier in those with diabetes—even children (with type 1). Cataracts can be easily treated, however; the doctor just removes the clouded lens and replaces it with a permanent contact lens.

The Least You Need to Know

- People with diabetes have a much higher risk of developing eye conditions that could lead to blindness.

- Diabetic retinopathy is the most common cause of blindness in people under 65.

- Regular eye exams and early diagnosis can prevent any significant vision loss from diabetic retinopathy.

- People with diabetes are also more likely to have glaucoma, and tend to develop cataracts earlier, than those without the disease.

Chapter 18

Your Kidneys: Hidden Gems Worth Keeping Healthy

In This Chapter

- The link between diabetes and kidney disease
- A healthy kidney
- The effect of diabetes on your kidneys
- Managing kidney disease
- When your kidneys fail

With only 11,000 people, Gila River in Arizona is one of the smallest communities in the United States, if not *the* smallest—to have its own *dialysis* center. Gila River is home to a Pima Indian tribe, and the Pimas have the highest rates of type 2 diabetes in the world. That fact attests to the terrible toll diabetes takes on your kidneys. They have rates of kidney failure 20 times higher than the general U.S. population, with diabetes to blame in 90 percent of the cases.

You may not be a Pima Indian, but if you have type 2 diabetes, your risk for serious kidney disease, called *nephropathy*, is many times higher than if you don't have diabetes. In fact, diabetes now accounts for about 45 percent of all cases of *end-stage renal disease (ESRD)*, in which the kidneys fail and you have to start on dialysis. People with diabetes also make up the fastest group of renal dialysis and kidney transplant patients in the country.

This chapter discusses what you need to know to stay out of that statistic.

MedLingo

Dialysis is a process by which a machine takes on the role of the kidneys, clearing the blood of toxins and other harmful substances.

Nephropathy is a form of kidney disease occurring in people with diabetes.

End-stage renal disease (ESRD) is when your kidneys are only working at less than 15 percent of their normal function. Typically, this is when dialysis begins.

Your Kidneys: Without Diabetes

Your kidneys are two purplish-brown, bean-shaped organs nestled against the middle back muscles on either side of your body. They are protected somewhat by the over-hang of the rib cage.

Their job is to maintain body fluids and salt balance, remove body wastes, and produce a hormone called *erythropoietin*, which directs the bone marrow to make red blood cells. With all this fluid and salt regulation, it should come as no surprise that they also play a major role in regulating blood pressure.

MedLingo

The kidneys produce a hormone called **erythropoietin**, which directs the production of red blood cells. **Glomeruli** are clusters of tiny blood vessels in the kidneys that filter blood.

In fact, if you have high blood pressure or diabetic retinopathy, you're much more likely to have kidney disease, too.

Think of the kidneys as a fine-mesh strainer. The "mesh" is actually called *glomeruli*, which are clusters of tiny blood vessels that filter your blood. It lets out water and some waste products and sends cleansed blood back through the circulatory system. Normal kidneys prevent protein from entering the urine; diseased kidneys don't.

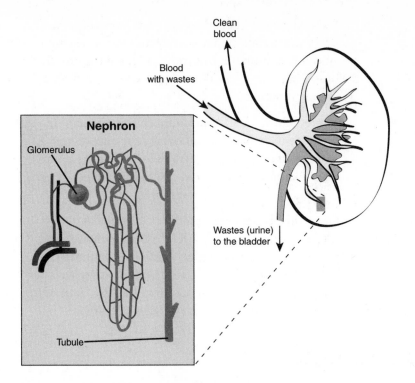

The Kidneys ©National Institute of Health

Your Kidneys: With Diabetes

Diabetic kidney disease, or diabetic nephropathy, is a microvascular disease, a disease of the small blood vessels. When you have diabetes, exposure to high levels of glucose for many years can create complicated changes in the nephrons. These changes cause the glomeruli, or "mesh" openings, to get larger, allowing protein molecules to escape.

Hence, people with diabetes often "spill" protein into their urine. The first protein that is spilled, and the one that remains the most common, is albumin. When only a small amount of it is excreted into the urine, it is called microalbuminuria. It is one of the earliest signs of kidney damage. That's why urine tests are such an important part of routine diabetes care.

In the early stages of kidney disease, lowering the blood sugar levels to near normal can reverse microalbuminuria, restoring normal kidney function. Getting high blood pressure back to normal can also help reverse microalbuminuria.

However, once the kidney damage has progressed beyond a certain point, as reflected by increasing amounts of albumin lost into urine, controlling the blood sugar and blood pressure alone won't improve kidney function.

Nonetheless, it's still very important to control blood pressure to reduce further damage to the kidney. The amount of albumin lost into the urine at the point where kidney damage is irreversible is called clinical proteinuria, or macroalbuminuria.

Once this damage occurs, the rest of your kidney's filters have to work extra hard to compensate. And, just as if you ran an engine at full speed all the time, eventually they also fail. Once your kidneys are operating at less than 15 percent of their capacity, you're diagnosed with ESRD and usually begin dialysis, and, if you're eligible, you join the kidney transplant list.

Recognizing Kidney Disease

Like diabetic retinopathy, there are no early symptoms of kidney disease. That's why regular testing is so important. The most commonly conducted tests for kidney disease are as follows:

- **Microalbumin.** This urine test, typically conducted either on a sample of urine collected in the morning or on the entire amount of urine collected over 24 hours, tests for very tiny amounts of the protein albumin in your urine. If the test is positive, you have microalbuminuria, which indicates that you're in the very early, yet reversible, phases of kidney disease.

- **Creatinine.** This blood test measures how well your kidneys excrete creatinine, one of the toxins your kidneys normally remove from the blood. If levels of blood creatinine are low, that's good. It means the kidneys are doing their job in clearing the blood of this waste product. If levels of blood creatinine are high, that's not so good, especially since creatinine levels in the blood don't start to increase until about 40 percent of kidney function is lost.

- **Glomerular Filtration Rate (GFR).** GFR is a more sensitive test and is one of the best ways to evaluate your kidney function and determine the stage of your kidney disease. This is a measure of how fast the creatinine is cleared from the blood. It's actually a calculation based on the results of your blood creatinine test, age, body size, and gender. The following table from the National Kidney Foundation shows how the GFR correlates with the stage of kidney disease.

Stages of Kidney Disease

Stage	Description	Glomerular Filtration Rate (GFR)*
At increased risk, but the presence of risk factors for kidney disease (e.g., diabetes, high blood pressure, family history, older age, certain ethnic groups, e.g., African-Americans)	No kidney damage	More than 90
1	Kidney damage (protein in the urine) and normal GFR	More than 90
2	Kidney damage and mild decrease in GFR	60 to 89
3	Moderate decrease in GFR	30 to 59
4	Severe decrease in GFR	15 to 29
5	Kidney failure (dialysis or kidney transplant needed)	Less than 15

*ml per min per 1.73 m^2 body surface area

> **Warning** _____
>
> If you experience any of the following physical symptoms, contact your doctor immediately. They could be signs of serious kidney disease:
>
> ♦ Leg swelling
> ♦ Loss of appetite and/or metallic taste in your mouth
> ♦ Less need for insulin or anti-diabetes pills
> ♦ Nausea and vomiting
> ♦ Weakness, paleness
> ♦ Severe itching

Managing Diabetic Nephropathy

Although there is no cure for diabetic nephropathy, there are ways to slow the progression of the disease. Specifically, you're going to have to control your blood pressure, control your high blood sugar, and change your diet. Once kidney disease starts, the most important of these three is to control your blood pressure.

Controlling High Blood Pressure

You know all about blood pressure from reading Chapter 16. There are two important things to understand here. The most important is that your blood pressure needs to be less than 130/80 mm Hg to slow the rate at which the kidneys lose function. If your blood creatinine is higher than normal, your blood pressure goal is even lower: 125/75 mm Hg. Studies find that reducing blood pressure to these levels can significantly slow the rate of kidney function loss.

Second, in Chapter 16 we talked about two classes of medications for lowering blood pressure: ACE (or angiotensin-converting enzyme inhibitors), and ARBs (or angiotensin receptor blockers). They're often prescribed for people with diabetes, particularly since many studies find they are more effective than any other antihypertensive drugs in slowing kidney damage. Unless there is a reason not to, you should be taking one of them.

This is also important because as someone with kidney disease, you're also more likely to develop cardiovascular disease on top of the already increased risk you have from your diabetes. Controlling your blood pressure is one important step in reducing that risk as well.

Controlling Blood Sugar

This second approach should come as no surprise. You already know that high blood sugar levels can damage your eyes and nerves, so of course it's going to affect your kidneys. Unfortunately, once you have clinical proteinuria, the horse may already be out of the barn. In other words, controlling your blood sugars at this point may not slow the loss of kidney function much. That's why we keep harping, nagging, kvetching over and over again about the importance of controlling blood sugar levels right from the get-go.

Following Your Diet

As we discussed in Chapter 16, a key part of any high blood pressure diet is reducing the amount of salt in your diet. There's also some evidence, as we've discussed before, that a high protein diet might result in kidney damage in people with diabetes, which is why some doctors recommend reducing the amount of protein in your diet if you have any nephropathy.

> **Bet You Didn't Know**
>
> If you are diagnosed with ESRD, you can receive coverage under Medicare, regardless of your age. Medicare covers more than 92 percent of dialysis patients and 90 percent of kidney transplant patients.

When Your Kidneys Fail

Although the percentage of people with ESRD who also have diabetes is very high (almost half of people starting dialysis now have kidney failure due to diabetes), ESRD or kidney failure occurs in a minority of people with diabetes and takes decades to develop. If your kidney function gets to stage 3, your doctor will probably refer you to a kidney specialist, called a *nephrologist*.

If you do reach stage 5 or ESRD, however, you have two options: kidney dialysis, either *hemodialysis* or *peritoneal dialysis*, or kidney transplant.

MedLingo

There are two types of dialysis: **hemodialysis,** in which you are hooked up to a machine for several hours three times a week, and **peritoneal dialysis,** in which a special solution inserted into your abdomen clears the blood of toxins without your having to be connected to a machine. When you have kidney disease, a **nephrologist**, a doctor trained in diseases of the kidneys, monitors your care.

Hemodialysis: An Artificial Kidney

Dialysis isn't fun and it isn't pretty, but it is a lifesaver. Without it, you would simply get sicker and sicker as more and more toxins built up in your blood, and eventually you'd die unless you got a kidney transplant.

When you're undergoing *hemodialysis*, you go to a kidney dialysis center. There are more than 3,600 dialysis centers in the United States, most of them located separate from hospitals.

This form of dialysis uses an artificial kidney called a *hemodialyzer* to remove waste and extra chemicals and fluid from your blood.

You'll usually need hemodialysis three times a week, and each session lasts from three to four hours. You also have to adhere to a strict schedule of hemodialysis, usually a Monday-Wednesday-Friday schedule or a Tuesday-Thursday-Saturday schedule, with a morning, evening, or afternoon shift.

You may be able to do your own dialysis at home, however, if you have a family member or friend to help provide the treatment.

A type of hemodialysis called *high-flux dialysis*, or high-efficiency dialysis, enables the removal of larger molecules and takes about 25 percent less time than hemodialysis. Ask your nephrologist if you're a candidate for this form.

Getting Started with Hemodialysis

Before you can begin hemodialysis, doctors need to create some form of access to your blood system, called *vascular access*. This is usually done weeks or even months before you begin dialysis.

There are three basic kinds of vascular accesses for hemodialysis:

◆ **Arteriovenous (AV) fistula.** A surgeon connects an artery directly to a vein, usually in the forearm. This, in turn, results in more blood flowing into the vein, strengthening the vein and making it grow larger and stronger. This is the preferred method of access.

◆ **AV graft.** This is used if you have small veins that won't develop into a fistula. The surgeon implants a synthetic tube under the skin in your arm and connects the artery to the nearest large vein, even though it may not be right next to the artery.

◆ **Venous catheter.** Used if your kidney disease progressed quickly and you don't have time for a permanent vascular access before starting hemodialysis. The surgeon inserts a tube, or catheter, with two holes in the side. This allows blood to be withdrawn through one of the holes, go through the hemodialyzer machine, and return to the blood stream through the second hole. The catheter is inserted into a vein in your neck, chest, or leg near the groin.

Peritoneal Dialysis: Mobile Dialysis

This form of dialysis provides more flexibility in terms of when and how you have your dialysis, but it requires more of you. In peritoneal dialysis, or PD, a soft tube called a catheter is used to fill your abdomen with a cleansing liquid called *dialysis solution*.

The dialysis solution exchanges with the liquid part of the blood. In this manner, the toxins or waste products from your blood pass through the lining of your abdomen into the dialysis solution in the abdominal cavity. These wastes then leave your body when the dialysis solution is drained.

The entire process of draining and filling is called an *exchange* and takes about 30 to 40 minutes. A typical schedule calls for four exchanges a day, each with a *dwell time* (the amount of time the solution is in your abdomen) of four to six hours.

Although there are different forms of PD, the most common form, continuous ambulatory peritoneal dialysis (CAPD), doesn't require a machine and you can walk around with the dialysis solution in your abdomen. Other types work while you sleep.

MedLingo

A **dialysis solution** is used during peritoneal dialysis to pull wastes into your abdominal cavity, after which the fluid is drained out. The process of draining and filling is called an **exchange,** and the fluid typically remains in your abdominal cavity for four to six hours, called the **dwell time.** The most common form of PD is called **continuous ambulatory peritoneal dialysis (CAPD)**.

Time for a New Kidney

Although kidney dialysis can add years to your life, it's just not as good as the real thing. People on long-term dialysis often wind up with thinning and weaker bones, itching, anemia, sleep disorders, and joint pain. Eventually, they usually need a kidney transplant if they can get one.

As a matter of fact, doctors prefer that patients with ESRD get kidney transplants rather than undergo dialysis at all. Even though it means you have to take strong drugs to protect your new kidney, a kidney transplant seems to have better results than dialysis.

This is no easy thing to accomplish. As of mid-2005, 65,000 people were on the waiting list for a kidney transplant. The good news is that a growing number of kidney transplants today come from living donors, relatives, friends, or even incredibly generous strangers, who volunteer to give up one healthy kidney (you only need one to survive) to help you out.

> **Bet You Didn't Know**
>
> According to the National Kidney Foundation, about 88.3 percent of the kidneys transplanted from cadavers (people who had died recently) are still functioning well at one year after surgery. The results are even better for kidneys transplanted from living donors. One year after surgery, 94 percent of these kidneys were still functioning well.

In fact, the National Kidney Foundation notes that of the 15,991 single kidney transplants performed in 2004, 6,642 (42 percent) were from living donors and the rest were from cadaveric donors (people who had recently died).

Today, it's never been easier to donate a kidney. It used to be that the donor had to have the same blood type as the recipient. But now, thanks to new processes provided at certain transplant centers, a recipient can receive a kidney from a donor of a different blood type.

Urinary Tract Infections

In addition to nephropathy, you also have to watch out for urinary tract infections (UTIs), which start in the bladder but can become much more serious by traveling back up into the kidney. As someone with diabetes, you're about five times more likely to get them than someone without the disease, particularly if you're a woman. Also, they can be more serious and last longer than the same infection in someone without diabetes, and over time, they can cause kidney damage if the infection travels upstream into the kidneys.

Common signs of a urinary tract infection include a frequent urge to urinate and a painful, burning feeling in the area of the bladder or urethra (the tube that goes from the bladder to the outside) during urination. You may also feel like you have the flu—tired, shaky, washed out—and feel pain even when you're not urinating. The urine itself may look milky or cloudy, even reddish if blood is present. If you have a fever, then the infection has probably backed up from the bladder and hit your kidneys.

UTIs and kidney infections are typically treated with antibiotics. If you're prone to UTIs several times a year, your doctor may want to put you on antibiotics *prophylactically*, to prevent infections. Most likely, however, he or she will call in a prescription for you after talking to you on the phone.

MedLingo

Prophylactically is any medical treatment or procedure performed to prevent a disease.

Angiogram is a medical procedure in which contrast dye is injected into your blood stream, enabling doctors (radiologists) to clearly see blood flow through many parts of your body.

Warning

People with diabetes are more likely to experience complications and even harm their kidney function when they undergo tests that require the injection of a dye into the blood stream, like *angiograms*. In one study, researchers found that the risk of kidney damage from such dyes, called contrast agents, was 50 to 90 percent higher for those who already had severe kidney problems, and 9 to 40 percent higher for those with mild to moderate kidney problems.

The Least You Need to Know

◆ You have a much higher risk of kidney disease because you have diabetes.

◆ You should have regular tests of your kidney function.

◆ The best way to prevent or slow the progression of kidney disease is by managing your blood pressure and blood glucose levels, and following a low-salt, low-protein diet.

◆ If you develop end-stage renal disease, you will need dialysis or a kidney transplant.

◆ You have a higher risk for urinary tract infections, which can lead to kidney damage.

Chapter 19

Navigating Your Way Through the Diabetic Neuropathies

In This Chapter

- ◆ Your risk of nerve damage
- ◆ Understanding your nervous system
- ◆ Various forms of diabetic neuropathy
- ◆ Prevention and early diagnosis
- ◆ Treatment for pain and beyond

When you stub your toe, it hurts. When you have to go the bathroom, you feel a sense of pressure. When you touch something hot, it burns. All these sensations rely on your *nervous system* to transmit impulses from your skin, bladder, and muscles to your brain, and vice versa. Even the ability of your blood vessels to constrict and expand, and of your heart to beat at a healthy pace, are related to your nervous system.

But when you have diabetes, your body's ability to feel, to sense, to send many of the minute-to-minute sensations and signals that make life possible may eventually become diminished as part of a group of conditions lumped under the term *diabetic neuropathy*. Conversely, you may experience excruciating pain as your *nerves* go into overdrive, making even the slightest touch of the sheet on your feet feel like being raked over coals.

MedLingo

The **nervous system** provides sensory and control mechanisms through a network of **nerve** cells, a collection of fibers that transmit signals to and from the brain and spinal cord to other parts of the body.

Diabetic neuropathy is the umbrella term for several conditions that affect the nervous system in people with diabetes. **Automatic neuropathy** is a form of neuropathy that affects the automatic nervous system, the part that controls functions such as breathing, digestion, heartbeat, and certain smooth muscles.

Diabetic Neuropathy Unplugged

Put simply, diabetic neuropathy is a nerve disorder in which the nerves become damaged. It generally occurs over years, and may affect numerous body systems, including the digestive tract, sexual organs, and urinary tract, as well as your feet, legs, and hands.

Diabetic neuropathy is one of the most common complications of diabetes regardless of the type of diabetes. It eventually affects 60 to 70 percent of all people with diabetes. It accounts for 50 to 75 percent of nontraumatic amputations (those that aren't related to accidents), increasing the overall risk of amputation up to 12-fold. In fact, neuropathy is the underlying reason for 87 percent of the 85,000 amputations in the lower extremities performed in the United States each year.

Neuropathy is a secretive disease, working its damage for years with no symptoms. Then, symptoms either come on gradually, or attack out of the blue. Sometimes, the symptoms seem to suddenly disappear, only to return later. In other cases, they disappear for good, but, as we'll talk about later, that's not necessarily a good thing; it may mean your nerves are so damaged that you can't feel anything anymore. And it doesn't matter if you have type 1 or type 2 diabetes; diabetic neuropathy is just as common in each.

> **CAUTION**
>
> **Warning**
>
> If you're cold in the winter, get an extra blanket, but stay away from electric blankets and heating pads. If you have neuropathy, you could burn yourself with these items because you might not be able to feel how hot they are. The same goes for hot baths. Since your feet are much more likely to become numb than your hands, and your hands much less so than your upper arms, if you have neuropathy, test the water with your elbow.

Understanding the Nervous System

First, here is some basic background information on the nervous system. Your nervous system is divided into three parts:

♦ The central nervous system (CNS), consisting of the brain and spinal cord

♦ The peripheral nervous system, consisting of all the nerves that branch out from the brain and spinal cord and go to the arms and legs

♦ The autonomic nervous system, consisting of the nerves that affect functions of the body you can't consciously control, like breathing, blood pressure, and digestion

There are two primary types of peripheral nerves:

♦ Sensory nerves, which take messages from your body to your brain and spinal cord; e.g., when you stub your toe, sensory nerves in your toe relay the stub to your brain, which registers pain.

♦ Motor nerves, which carry signals from your brain and spinal cord to your muscles, enabling you to walk, move, spin, run, jump, etc.

Diabetic neuropathy affects the peripheral and autonomic nerves.

Neuropathy by Any Other Name

There are numerous forms of neuropathy, all with their own symptoms and names, and we list most below. But on a big picture level there are three general types of neuropathies.

The most common is *peripheral neuropathy*. This form affects the nerves that go to the feet and, sometimes, the hands. The first symptom is usually pain, a burning, tingly feeling that can become quite nasty.

Eventually the pain disappears and is replaced by numbness. This doesn't mean the nerves are better. This lack of feeling occurs because the nerves are now dead, so you can't feel much at all. This increases the danger of foot ulcers, which we talk more about in Chapter 20.

The second type of diabetic neuropathy is *autonomic neuropathy*, which affects the nerves you can't consciously control like those that control breathing, control your heart rate, and direct the actions of smooth muscles like those in the digestive system. Damage to the autonomic nerves occurs over long periods without any symptoms. When symptoms do appear, they differ, depending upon which organs are most affected.

The third type of diabetic neuropathy, called *acute-onset neuropathy*, or *focal neuropathy*, usually involves just one nerve. In contrast to the gradual onset of the first two types, the symptoms in this form come on fast.

This form is associated with pain as well as weakness of the muscles affected by the nerves. The good news is that the pain and muscle weakness is temporary, and everything usually returns to normal within a few months to a year.

MedLingo

Peripheral neuropathy affects the feet, and, less commonly, the hands on both sides of your body. At any one time, about 25 to 30 percent of people with type 2 diabetes will complain of pain in their feet due to peripheral neuropathy. The pain usually disappears over time because the nerve damage gets worse and the feet become numb. After many years of diabetes, 60 to 70 percent of diabetic patients will develop peripheral neuropathy.

Autonomic neuropathy affects several organ systems. About one-third of people with type 2 diabetes develop automatic neuropathy, although symptoms don't usually appear until later in life. Many people never have any of the symptoms.

Acute-onset neuropathy, or **focal neuropathy**, usually involves just one nerve, and symptoms come on fast. It is usually quite painful. Fortunately, this type of neuropathy is not too common.

Specific Forms of Neuropathy

Depending on which part of the nervous system is involved, neuropathy can take many different forms.

- **Peripheral neuropathy.** This is the most frequently diagnosed type of neuropathy and usually affects both feet. It is behind 85 percent of amputations of the toes, feet and legs because it may lead to foot ulcers, which, in turn, may result in *gangrene* followed by blood poisoning. When the feet become numb, you can't feel minor traumas and pain, and so you might not protect your feet from injury, which could result in severe damage.

- **Femoral neuropathy** (also called diabetic amyotrophy). This is an acute-onset neuropathy affecting the thigh muscles. It can be extremely painful. It usually affects both sides, and is associated with weakness of the thigh muscles. Because it can take up to a year or more to go away, the thigh muscles sometimes shrink. This form is most common in people with type 2 diabetes.

- **Gastroparesis.** A form of autonomic neuropathy affecting the stomach that prevents it from emptying normally. Instead, food remains in the stomach for a long time (often hours). Symptoms include feeling full after only eating a little bit, feeling bloated after eating, nausea, abdominal cramps, and vomiting (sometimes undigested food many hours after you've eaten).

- **Diabetic diarrhea.** This form of autonomic neuropathy affects functioning of the small intestine, which can cause you to pass unformed stools. Because nerve damage may weaken the ring of muscle in the *rectum*

MedLingo

Gangrene results when tissue doesn't get enough oxygenated blood, and dies. The tissue looks dark and eventually black. There is no treatment to reverse it once it reaches the black stage. It must be amputated. If it is a small area, for instance part of a toe, it might fall off by itself (auto-amputation). Otherwise a surgeon has to amputate the tissue.

Warning

If you're taking insulin, gastroparesis can be a real problem. It can cause hypoglycemia because there's a mismatch between the action of insulin after injection, the delayed entry of food into the intestine, and the appearance of glucose in the blood from the food.

MedLingo

The **rectum** is the final part of the large intestine that controls bowel movements.

that controls bowel movements, stool may leak out, especially while sleeping. This is called fecal incontinence, or an inability to control your bowel movements. Automatic neuropathy of the small intestine is actually more likely to lead to constipation. A common pattern is alternating diarrhea and constipation.

♦ **Bladder neuropathy.** This form of automatic neuropathy occurs when the bladder nerves no longer respond normally to pressure as the bladder fills with urine, so you can't completely empty your bladder. Thus, some urine continually stays in the bladder, leading to urinary tract infections.

♦ **Postural hypotension.** This is a form of autonomic neuropathy that results in low blood pressure when standing, leading to dizziness and fainting. Normally, when you stand up, blood vessels in your legs constrict, sending more blood to the heart, which can then pump the blood to the brain. In postural hypotension, the neuropathy has affected the nerves that regulate blood vessel contraction in the legs when you stand up. So too little blood gets to the heart to be pumped to the brain, causing dizziness and faintness.

♦ **Charcot joint.** Also called neuropathic arthropathy, this form of peripheral neuropathy occurs when the bones in the feet fracture and the foot becomes misaligned (that is, not lined up the way they should be). We think that this occurs because there is no feeling in the feet. Thus, repeated traumas that you can't feel result in broken bones, and your muscles no longer properly support your foot. Walking only makes this condition worse.

♦ **Unilateral foot drop.** This form of acute-onset neuropathy occurs when you can't pick up your foot because a nerve in your leg is damaged, so you drag your foot.

♦ **Erectile dysfunction or impotence.** We talked about this in Chapter 13, but it's important to understand that it's most often caused by autonomic neuropathy.

♦ **Cranial nerve neuropathy.** This form affects the nerves that control the movement of your eyeballs. Since only one side is affected, the eyeballs can't move together, resulting in double vision. There is also pain behind the affected eye. Usually, it gets better on its own within a few weeks to a few months.

♦ **Gangrene** results when tissue doesn't get enough oxygenated blood, and dies.

♦ **Femoral neuropathy, also called diabetic amyotrophy,** is an extremely painful form of neuropathy affecting the thigh muscles, usually on both legs.

◆ **Gastroparesis** is a form of autonomic neuropathy affecting the stomach that prevents it from emptying normally.

◆ **Diabetic diarrhea** is a form of autonomic neuropathy affecting the functioning of the small intestine. Sometimes peripheral neuropathy has also weakened the ring of muscle in the **rectum**, the final part of the large intestine, that controls bowel movements, resulting in **fecal incontinence**, in which stool leaks out, especially while sleeping.

◆ **Bladder neuropathy** is a form of automatic neuropathy that occurs when the bladder nerves no longer respond normally to pressure.

◆ **Postural hypotension** is a form of autonomic neuropathy that results in low blood pressure when standing, leading to fainting and dizziness.

◆ **Charcot joint,** or **neuropathic arthropathy**, occurs when the bones in the feet fracture because of repeated unnoticed trauma and the foot becomes misaligned.

◆ **Unilateral foot drop** occurs when you can't pick up your foot because of a damaged nerve in the leg.

◆ **Erectile dysfunction** is often caused by damage to the nerves that control the entrance and trapping of blood in the penis.

◆ **Cranial neuropathy** affects the nerves that move the eyeballs.

What's Going On?

So why the nerve damage? We're not sure. Although there are several theories, one possible reason is long-term damage from *glycation*, the result of high glucose levels. With high blood sugar levels, extra glucose sticks to proteins and other cellular structures, damaging them and leading to many diabetes-related complications, including neuropathy.

MedLingo

Glycation occurs when extra glucose sticks to proteins and other cellular structures as a result of long-term high blood sugar levels.

Easy-to-Miss Early Warning Signs

The first sign something's wrong? When your doctor hits your ankle with a little rubber-capped hammer and nothing happens. No jerking, no movement. Sometimes you also lose knee reflexes.

Other early symptoms include a slight tingling in your toes, followed by a burning sensation that interferes with your sleeping. After that, you may experience numbness and eventually lose feeling in your feet.

For instance, you may be unable to feel a pinprick, temperature change, or even light touch sensation on your feet. That's why it's so important to take good care of your feet and have regular foot exams, as we discuss in the next chapter. Because once you lose feeling in your feet, you run the risk of a severe injury or ulceration that could lead to gangrene and limb amputation.

Symptoms of various neuropathies include the following:

◆ Numbness, tingling, or pain in your toes, feet, legs, fingers, hands, or arms

◆ Insensitivity to pain or temperature

◆ Extreme sensitivity to touch, even a light touch

◆ Loss of balance and coordination

◆ Weakness in your feet or hand muscles

◆ Indigestion, nausea, or vomiting

◆ Diarrhea or constipation

◆ Dizziness or faintness when you rise from a sitting or lying position

◆ Problems urinating

◆ Erectile dysfunction or vaginal dryness

Diagnosing Diabetic Neuropathy

As with every other diabetes-related complication, prevention (keeping your blood sugars near normal) is the way to go when it comes to diabetic neuropathy. Early diagnosis and early treatment are also important, however, if neuropathy does occur. There are several ways to diagnose, or at least keep a close watch on, the development of neuropathies, including the following:

◆ **Regular foot exams.** You should have regular foot exams every few months during your routine office visits. The doctor should examine your feet for any cuts, blisters, ulcers, or other damage, as well as test the level of sensation, or feeling, in your foot, often with a nylon brush. We talk more about foot care in Chapter 20.

- ◆ **Neurological examination.** The doctor asks you certain questions, tests your reflexes, tests your eyeball motion, and measures sensation in your feet and legs maybe with a vibrating tuning fork and a pin.

Doctors typically perform the following two tests if there is some question as to whether your symptoms are really due to diabetic neuropathy.

- ◆ *Nerve conduction tests* evaluate how well your nerves conduct sensation. You receive a small shock to a nerve, and an image of the nerve conducting the electrical signal is displayed on a computer screen. Conduction slows as neuropathy develops.

- ◆ *Electromyographic examination* measures the response of your muscles to the small shock similarly to the nerve conduction test.

The following tests are not routine and are only performed under special circumstances.

- ◆ *Quantitative sensory testing (QST)*, to measure your sensitivity to temperature, touch, pressure, vibration, and pain

- ◆ X-rays, in the case of joint problems related to neuropathy

- ◆ Ultrasound, to evaluate the function of your bladder

- ◆ Cardiovascular testing, to evaluate the condition of the nerves controlling the heart

- ◆ Gastrointestinal tests, to measure how fast the stomach empties

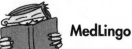

MedLingo

Nerve conduction tests evaluate how well your nerves conduct sensation, while **electromyographic examination** measures the response of your muscles to an electrical shock. **Quantitative sensory testing (QST)** measures your sensitivity to temperature, touch, pressure, vibration, and pain.

But It Hurts!

We know it does. Ironically, you'd think that if your nerves were being destroyed, you wouldn't feel anything. And, eventually in many patients, that's just what happens. But in the beginning of peripheral neuropathy, the nerves often seem to have switched into a permanent "on" position, sending pain signals to your brain even though there's no obvious reason for the pain.

In fact, a study published in the January 2005 issue of the journal *Diabetes Care* found a high prevalence of chronic pain among people with diabetes. The more pain people had to cope with, the poorer their diabetes management was likely to be, and the harder it was for them to follow exercise and eating plans and take their medication.

There are several options for pain relief, depending on the severity of the pain itself. These include the following:

◆ Acetaminophen (Tylenol).

◆ Nonsteroidal anti-inflammatory drugs (NSAIDs) such as aspirin, ibuprofen (Motrin), or naproxen (Aleve). Because these drugs slightly decrease blood flow to the kidneys, some doctors don't like to use them in people with diabetes who are already at risk for kidney disease.

◆ Topical creams to reduce pain that contain *capsaicin*, the same chemical that gives hot peppers their spiciness.

◆ Antidepressant medications such as amitriptyline, imipramine, and nortriptyline. In September 2004, the Food and Drug Administration approved Cymbalta (duloxetine) for managing diabetic peripheral neuropathic pain.

◆ Anticonvulsant medications such as Tegretol (carbamazepine) or Neurontin (gabapentin). In late 2004, the Food and Drug Administration approved the first treatment specifically for managing pain associated with diabetic peripheral neuropathy. Called Lyrica (pregabalin), it was expected to be available to patients sometime in 2005.

◆ Codeine, morphine, methadone, or other narcotics or opiates for short-term relief of severe pain.

> ### Bet You Didn't Know
>
> Cymbalta affects two major chemicals in the brain, norepinephrine and serotonin, which play a role in depression, mood, and pain perception. Studies find that Cybalta helps relieve the stabbing, burning, and shooting pain often associated with the disease.

> ### Sugar Sense
>
> Antidepressants may take several weeks or more to begin working, so be patient.

Other nonmedical treatments that seem to have some benefits for managing pain include:

◆ *Transcutaneous electronic nerve stimulation (TENS)*

◆ Hypnosis and biofeedback

- Relaxation training
- Acupuncture

MedLingo

- **Capsaicin** is a chemical that gives hot peppers their spiciness and can be used in a topical cream to reduce pain.
- **Serotonin** and **norepinephrine** are brain chemicals that play a role in depression and pain perception.
- **Transcutaneous electronic nerve stimulation (TENS)** is a drug-free therapy that works by inhibiting pain signals from reaching the brain.

Treating the Problem

As recently as 1994, an editorial in the medical journal *The Lancet* noted that, "all we can do for diabetic neuropathy is make the diagnosis and commiserate with the patient."

Thankfully, that's no longer the case.

Today, in addition to the above-mentioned treatments for pain, there are numerous medications and lifestyle changes that can help reduce the disability and symptoms resulting from various nephropathies. For instance ...

- Tightly control your blood sugars. Studies find that tightly controlled blood glucose levels not only delay and possibly prevent the onset of neuropathies, but can also reduce the initial pain that patients experience.

- If you have gastroparesis, eat small, frequent, low-fat meals with less fiber. This will reduce the nausea, bloating, abdominal cramps, and vomiting that often accompany this neuropathy.

Bet You Didn't Know

Drugs used to treat the symptoms of gastroparesis include *prokinetic agents,* drugs that make the muscles of the stomach contract to expel food. Common drugs used for this condition include Reglan (metoclopramide), Motilium (domperidone) (available in Canada) and erythromycin (an antibiotic).

◆ For neuropathic hypotension, get up slowly; don't quickly go from lying to standing, but stay in the sitting position for about a minute before standing. If that doesn't work, try wearing support stockings. This compresses blood vessels in your legs, sending blood back to the heart and preventing that lightheadedness when standing.

Your doctor may prescribe some medications, including the steroid, 9-fluorohydrocortisone, the blood pressure medication Catapres (clonidine), ProAmatine, (midodrine), or Sandostatin (octreotide), as well as supplemental salt.

◆ Creams and other emollients can soothe and protect dry, cracked skin on your feet and hands, preventing infections that could lead to ulcers and gangrene.

Warning

If you have neuropathic hypotension, skip hot baths. The heat further dilates blood vessels, making it difficult to increase the blood flow to the brain when you stand up to get out, increasing your risk of slipping and falling.

◆ If you're having bladder problems related to neuropathy, you'll be taught to "massage" or palpate your bladder when it's full to help you start urinating. To do this, press the abdomen just above your pubic bone to start the flow of urine. You may also learn to catheterize yourself, in which you insert a small tube through your urethra into the bladder to empty the bladder. Some medications are available, including bethanechol or Cardura (doxazosin).

The Least You Need to Know

◆ As someone with diabetes, you are likely to develop one or more neuropathies, or nerve damage.

◆ There are numerous forms of neuropathy, some painful, that can affect every part of your body from your feet and joints to your blood pressure, heartbeat, and ability to urinate.

◆ Tight blood sugar control can prevent and improve neuropathies early on, but not after they are fully developed.

◆ There are numerous medical and lifestyle treatments for the various forms of neuropathy, but no cure.

20

Focusing on the Externals

In This Chapter

- ◆ Taking care of your feet
- ◆ Medicare and your feet
- ◆ Taking care of your skin
- ◆ Taking care of your mouth

When you have diabetes, tiny little problems can quickly turn into major medical complications. Take a blister on the back of your heel, for instance. If you have some neuropathy, and don't realize it's there, it could easily become infected, possibly resulting in the amputation of your foot. A failure to floss your teeth could lead to serious gum disease, resulting in tooth loss. And ignore your weight and blood sugar for too long, and you could end up with disfiguring and uncomfortable skin conditions.

In diabetes, as with most things in life, it's the little things that matter. Take care of them, and the big things will take care of themselves. So in this chapter, we're going to focus on three key areas: your feet, your teeth (and gums), and your skin.

Focusing on the Feet

As you read in Chapter 19, diabetes is the leading cause of limb amputation in the country. A major reason? Foot ulcers that get out of control.

The greatest contributor to foot ulcers is peripheral neuropathy. Because it diminishes your ability to feel injuries, peripheral neuropathy increases your risk of foot ulcers sevenfold.

Another cause is too much pressure on the plantar area, the ball of the foot, often due to joint or bone problems. Other contributing factors include foot deformities and trauma to the foot, and even just ill-fitting shoes. One study of 669 people with a foot ulcer found that 21 percent of ulcers resulted from shoes rubbing against the foot, 11 percent from injuries (primarily falls), and 4 percent from cutting toenails (more on that later). Plus, after you've had an ulcer, it doesn't take much to make that ulcer return.

MedLingo

Gangrene refers to the death of body tissue, usually from a loss of blood flow.

Just because you have an ulcer doesn't necessarily mean you're going to lose your foot. But because people with diabetes are also more likely to have peripheral vascular disease, in which the arteries in the legs are clogged, and problems with their body's ability to heal wounds (if blood sugar is too high), it's often difficult to heal an ulcer. This can result in *gangrene.* So good preventive foot care is critical.

Sugar Sense

Consider adding a podiatrist to your healthcare team. A few studies looking at the benefits of foot specialty care found that people with diabetes receiving podiatric care had fewer deep foot ulcers than those who didn't, and fewer hospital admission days. Studies also find that the more often you receive routine and follow-up foot care, the less likely you are to develop an ulcer and require an amputation.

Keeping Your Tootsies Healthy

The first step toward healthy feet is prevention. That means …

 ◆ Understanding your risk for foot ulcers. If you've had diabetes more than 10 years, had previous foot ulcerations, had a previous amputation (even a toe), have HgA1c levels greater than 9 percent, and have problems with your vision, you're much more likely to develop foot ulcers and other such complications.

◆ Receiving an annual foot exam from your physician. This should include assessing the structure of your foot, how it works while walking, blood flow, and skin condition. If you have any existing foot conditions, or meet the criteria for higher risk described above, you'll need additional exams throughout the year.

◆ Bathing your feet every day with warm water and soap, and rinsing and thoroughly drying, particularly between your toes.

◆ Trimming your toenails with a nail file, *not* with scissors or clippers. File straight across, with a curve at the edge to avoid bothering the next toe. If you have any foot problems, don't try this yourself; instead, see a *podiatrist* for nail care.

◆ Having any corns or calluses professionally removed.

◆ Using a moisturizing cream on dry feet, but avoiding the spaces between the toes.

◆ Inspecting your feet daily for any cuts, red spots, warm spots, calluses, corns, ingrown toenails, discoloration, or any other abnormalities. Use a mirror so that you can see everywhere!

◆ Looking out for calluses. These hard, roughened areas on the bottom of your feet are markers of increased pressure on the foot. The increased pressure interferes with the blood supply. Thus, ulcers can be lurking below the callus. By keeping calluses thin, you reduce the increased pressure and the chance for an ulcer. You also need to find out why there is increased pressure on that part of the foot.

◆ Always wearing shoes. Don't ever go barefoot, even in the pool or at the beach. A tiny splinter or cut from stepping on a sharp shell could cause a serious ulcer. Walking on a hot surface that you can't feel can lead to burns and other major problems.

Warning _____

Don't try and remove any corns or calluses yourself with over-the-counter treatments; this could cause a serious injury.

MedLingo _____

A **podiatrist** is a specialist in the care of the feet.

Orthotics are devices used to support, align, prevent, or correct deformities or to improve the function of parts of the body, such as the foot.

You should also try to maintain healthy blood sugar control, quit smoking (if you haven't already), and consider specially made shoes and *orthotics* if you have a high risk of foot ulcers.

One of the most important things you can do when it comes to foot health is to buy and wear the proper shoes.

- ◆ Make sure your shoes are comfortable and provide plenty of room for your toes to move. If they cause blisters or calluses, they're not right for you.

- ◆ Always try on shoes with the socks you intend to wear with them. Go shoe shopping late in the day, when your feet are at their largest.

- ◆ Leave Internet shoe shopping to people without diabetes. You need to try on your shoes in the store to make sure they fit properly.

- ◆ Measure both feet every time you go shoe shopping. You may find that one foot is larger than the other. Plus, as we age, our feet tend to get bigger.

- ◆ Go for quality; that means real leather and other natural materials that "breathe," not synthetics.

- ◆ If the shoes aren't comfortable in the store, don't buy them. They're not going to "break in" without some discomfort and potential harm to your feet; you don't need that.

- ◆ When you get a new pair of shoes, wear them for just a couple of hours a day for the first couple of weeks, carefully examining your feet after each wearing for any signs of damage.

- ◆ Go for flat shoes over high heels, and lace-ups over slip-ons.

Detecting Foot Problems Early

As we said earlier, it's important that your doctor evaluate your feet on a regular basis to catch any problems before they develop into something serious. That means …

- ◆ Screening for loss of sensation. This gets back to keeping a close eye on the development of any neuropathy. Insist that your doctor screen you during each visit for diabetes.

- ◆ Screening for high "plantar pressure." To get fancy about it, your podiatrist can screen you with special mats and instruments designed to measure the pressure inside your shoes.

◆ Screening for peripheral vascular disease. This usually involves feeling for pulses at several areas in the leg and feet and comparing your blood pressure in your arm to that in your ankle.

Medicare and Foot Care

Medicare, the federally funded health insurance program that covers those 65 and older, people with disabilities, or those with end-stage renal disease, offers a therapeutic shoe program for people with diabetes. The program pays 80 percent of a specified amount for one pair of shoes and up to three pairs of molded innersoles per year.

To qualify, you must be under a comprehensive diabetes treatment plan and have one or more of the following:

◆ A history of partial or complete amputation of the foot

◆ A history of previous foot ulceration

◆ A history of pre-ulcerative calluses

◆ Peripheral neuropathy with some evidence of callus formation

◆ A foot deformity

◆ Poor circulation

You'll need a prescription for the shoes from a podiatrist or qualified doctor, and the shoes must be fitted and provided by a doctor or other individual like a *pedorthist, orthotist,* or *prosthetist.*

Coverage is limited to one of the following per calendar year:

◆ One pair of depth-inlay shoes and three pairs of inserts, or

◆ One pair of custom-molded shoes (including inserts) if you can't wear depth-inlay shoes because of a foot deformity, and two additional pairs of inserts within the calendar year.

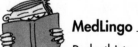

MedLingo

Pedorthists, orthotists, or **prosthetists** are individuals skilled in the manufacture of foot orthotics.

Treating Foot Ulcers

Unfortunately, there's no magic pill you can take to treat a foot ulcer. Instead, you have to follow a multidisciplinary approach. Resting and elevating the foot—i.e., *staying off it*—is the first step (forgive the pun) and by far the most important thing you can do to heal the ulcer. Failing to stay off of your foot is the most common reason for foot ulcers that don't heal, resulting in amputations.

Also check your footwear; if you're not sure whether it's appropriate, bring it with you to your doctor's office and let your doctor check it.

Your doctor, or more likely your podiatrist, may also recommend several footwear devices designed to keep pressure off the plantar area of the foot (where most ulcers occur) while you heal.

Now, here's the not-so-pleasant part. Your doctor may have to *debride*, or scrape away, dead tissue from within and around the ulcer, trying to keep the area clean and free of infection. Most of the time, your foot has lost so much sensation that this doesn't hurt very much. If it does, keep in mind that it hurts less than an amputation.

MedLingo

Debride means to scrape away dead tissue.

Warning

Don't soak your feet if you have an ulcer. You could inadvertently burn your foot if the water is too hot.

Don't be tempted by any over-the-counter creams or ointments; even most prescription preparations aren't very much use. Instead, keeping the foot warm and protected from contamination seems to be the best way to heal ulcers. If the ulcer isn't too bad, you may be asked to do some debriding yourself by using "wet to dry" dressing changes.

You place a wet gauze over the ulcer, let it dry, and when it's removed, it takes away some dead tissue. By doing this several times a day, you keep the base of the ulcer clean and help it heal. (Ulcers heal from the bottom up, not from the top down.)

Bet You Didn't Know

There is one pharmaceutical product approved for foot ulcers: a growth factor called Regranex (becaplermin). Growth factors stimulate repair of the tissue at the injury site, helping form the basis for wound healing. Additionally, there are bioengineered skin (Apligraf) and human skin (Dermagraft) substances that can enhance healing. Believe it or not, they're derived from the foreskins of newborn penises.

If your foot isn't healing, you may need to see a vascular surgeon to evaluate the blood flow to the wound. Without healthy blood flow, it's hard for the ulcer to heal. Also, if there's any infection, expect your doctor to start you on antibiotics, both oral and topical (in cream).

However, only about 15 percent of ulcers that don't heal are due to poor blood flow. Most of the time, the problem is related to the fact that the patient keeps walking on it.

Taking Care of Your Teeth

As someone with diabetes, you have about twice the risk of developing gum disease, also called *gingivitis* or *periodontal disease*, as someone without diabetes. In fact, about one third of those with diabetes have such severe gum disease that their teeth begin to come loose from their gums.

Gum disease results from bacteria growing between your teeth and gums. Some studies suggest that it may contribute to the development of type 2 diabetes to begin with, and other studies suggest that periodontal disease affects your control of existing diabetes. Conversely, treating periodontal disease can be difficult if blood sugars are high. And smoking makes the problem worse.

So preventing and controlling periodontal disease is a critical part of your diabetes management program.

MedLingo

Gingivitis, also called **periodontal disease,** results from infections caused by bacteria growing between your teeth and gums.

Beyond Brushing

We're going to assume that you're doing the bare minimum: brushing your teeth at least twice a day with a quality toothpaste. Well, how about upping that to three times a day or after every meal?

And what about flossing? Sure, flossing is a pain, but with all the flavored flosses and cool flossing implements out there these days, it's ever so much easier to floss. Flossing after every meal is what dentists recommend.

Sugar Sense

Examine your teeth and gums every day for any redness or swelling, bleeding of the gums, loose teeth, receding gums, and increased spacing between your teeth. If you see any of these signs, visit your dentist as soon as possible. Another sign of gum disease is bad breath.

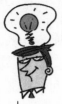

Sugar Sense

Having trouble remembering to floss after meals? Try these tips:

- ◆ Keep a container of dental floss in your car and floss at red lights.
- ◆ Keep a container of floss in your office on your desk, a handy reminder to floss after lunch.
- ◆ Toss a floss container into your pocket so it's always with you.

If you don't have any evidence of periodontal disease and your diabetes is well controlled, then you should see your dentist every six months for regular cleanings and have a full gum examination at least once a year.

But if your diabetes is poorly controlled, you need to be seen more often, sometimes as often as every three months if you have any existing evidence of gum disease.

Maintaining Beautiful (and Healthy) Skin

Another, less serious complication of diabetes affects the largest organ in your body: your skin. And, of course, skin conditions are linked to—ta da!—poor blood sugar control (are you sensing a pattern here?).

We've already talked about some skin-related diabetes complications, such as foot ulcers related to neuropathy. If you have peripheral vascular disease, the blood vessels that supply blood to your skin in your legs could also be affected, limiting the amount of oxygenated blood your skin receives and leading to hair loss and thin, shiny, cold skin.

And of course, without adequate blood flow, you don't have enough germ-fighting white blood cells to help prevent infections, or if one develops, to help fight it. This is one of many reasons you're more likely to develop skin-related infections.

Other diabetes-related skin conditions have a variety of tongue-twisting names that we're not going to burden you with here. Suffice it to say that they can result in thickened and/or darkened patches of skin; sores on the lower part of your legs; shiny round or oval lesions of thin skin on your legs that can itch and burn; thick, waxy, tight skin on your toes, fingers, and hands; or yellow, waxy, pea-like bumps on your skin that result from extremely high levels of triglycerides. Pretty gross, huh?

You're also prone to develop diabetic blisters, bacterial infections, and fungal infections of the skin (including jock itch, athlete's foot, and ringworm). Also, fungal infections of the toenails (causing thickened and discolored nails) are more common in people with diabetes.

Although a dermatologist can treat many of these conditions with medications, the best treatment (and prevention) is to maintain healthy blood sugar levels.

The Least You Need to Know

◆ Good foot care is critical to avoiding foot ulcers that could lead to amputation.

◆ You should have your feet professionally examined at least once a year, and you should examine them for ulcers, cuts, bruises, etc., on a daily basis.

◆ Good-fitting, comfortable shoes are very important for people with diabetes.

◆ You should brush your teeth at least twice a day, and floss at least daily, to avoid gum disease.

◆ Good blood sugar control will help reduce your risk of disfiguring and uncomfortable skin disorders.

Part 5

A Glimpse into the Future

This section might be the shortest of the five, but it's the most important. You learn in Chapter 21 how you can participate in the quest for a cure and better treatments for diabetes through clinical trials. Chapter 22 wraps up the book with a hopeful look into the future both in terms of treatments and a possible cure.

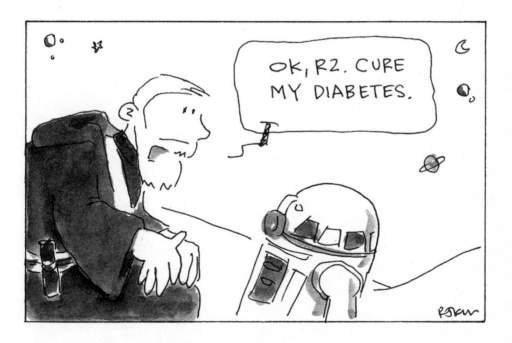

21

Moving Research Forward: Clinical Trials

In This Chapter

- Clinical trials and what they mean to you
- Types of clinical trials
- Phases of clinical trials
- Joining a clinical trial

If you're on insulin, you owe your life to a 14-year-old boy named Leonard Thompson. The child had type 1 diabetes (although back in 1922, no one knew there was more than one type of diabetes). He was dying because, back then, that's what you did if you had diabetes. But those famous researchers Frederic Banting and Charles Best (who later won the Nobel Prize for their discovery of insulin) injected the boy with pancreatic extracts, the first crude version of insulin, and he lived another 13 years.

Poor Lenny probably never knew it, but he participated in one of the first-ever diabetes-related clinical trials. In doing so, he (and the doctors who treated him) changed the world of diabetes forever. Pretty cool, huh? The cool part? You can do the same thing.

Clinical Trials: How Research Gets Done Today

Before the U.S. Food and Drug Administration (FDA) approves a drug or medical device for marketing in the United States, it must undergo extensive testing on animals and humans to prove that it is safe and effective. That requires clinical trials, and research studies involving hundreds, often thousands, of human volunteers. Such a trial is called a *treatment trial*.

Other types of clinical trials include the following:

♦ *Prevention trials*, which try to identify improved methods of preventing disease in people who have never had the disease or to prevent a disease from returning. For instance, a trial might be designed to see if tight blood glucose control can prevent retinopathy. In fact, numerous studies have proved just that point.

♦ *Diagnostic trials*, which try to find better tests or procedures to diagnose a particular disease or condition. For instance, experts might design a trial to test what level of HgA1c in people not known to have diabetes should be used to diagnose it.

♦ *Screening trials*, which identify the best way to detect certain diseases or health conditions. For instance, a trial might be designed to see if testing for microalbuminuria would identify people more likely to develop kidney failure. In fact, we know this is true because several trials did show this.

♦ *Quality-of-life trials* explore ways to improve the comfort and the quality of life for people with a chronic illness. For instance, a trial might be designed to see if people with diabetes are happier using an insulin pump or injectable insulin.

At any given time, there are thousands of clinical studies underway throughout the country, in private physician offices, academic medical centers, and community hospitals. And of those thousands, a large number involve some form of treatment, device, or observation related to diabetes.

You and Clinical Trials

All very well and good, you say. But what's this got to do with me? Well, it's very possible that you'll be asked at one point or another to participate in a clinical trial. It might be to test a new oral medication, to evaluate the effectiveness of a new glucose meter, or to determine whether a certain lifestyle change can reduce the risk of complications.

You could say no, but then you'd be turning your back on the opportunity to not only possibly improve your own health, but also improve the health of millions of others like you. There are also certain advantages to clinical trials:

◆ You may be eligible for free or at least reduced care and medications.

◆ You may be eligible for some financial compensation for your time.

◆ You may have access to treatments still considered experimental, but which may provide significant benefits.

◆ You have an opportunity to participate in the future of diabetes treatment.

The Downside to Clinical Trials

Okay, so there are some advantages. There are also some disadvantages. For instance, participating in a clinical trial means you might be exposed to more poking and prodding than if you continued with your routine care. It's also possible that you will experience a side effect of a new drug or device under investigation.

Clinical trials might also involve additional visits to the doctor, taking up more of your time and effort. Also, the trial might not cover all your care; your health insurance might have to pay for some, or you may have some out-of-pocket expenses.

And, finally, the biggest downside is that you might not actually get the "new" treatment being studied; instead, you might receive the old treatment, or a *placebo*, a "fake" treatment designed to mimic the look, taste, and feel of the treatment under evaluation.

MedLingo

A **placebo** is an inactive pill, liquid, or powder that has no treatment value. It is often used in clinical trials to compare with experimental treatments. No sick participant receives a placebo, however, if there is a known beneficial treatment.

Behind the Rhetoric of Clinical Trials

As with anything in medicine, clinical trials have their own vocabulary. If you're interested in joining a trial, it's important that you understand the lingo.

There are four primary levels, or phases, of clinical trials:

◆ **Phase I.** This is the first trial in humans. The number of people enrolled is small, usually only a dozen or so, and the goal is to evaluate the safety of the treatment in humans and the best way to give the treatment (orally, through injection, or through a nasal spray, for example). This phase normally enrolls completely healthy people, such as those *without* diabetes.

◆ **Phase II clinical trial.** This phase also evaluates the safety of a therapy, but begins to look at how well it works. One main goal is to determine the appropriate dosage for the treatment. Although these trials are larger, they still involve only about 100 or fewer people.

◆ **Phase III clinical trial.** This is the last phase that a drug undergoes before the pharmaceutical company submits paperwork to the FDA asking that the drug be approved. By the time a medication gets to this stage, the drug company has had some pretty favorable results and has determined that it's worth the fairly hefty investment it has to make to embark upon Phase III clinical trials. This is most likely the kind of clinical trial in which you would enroll. Generally, phase III clinical trials involve hundreds, if not thousands, of participants.

◆ **Phase IV clinical trial.** These trials occur after a drug is approved for marketing. The goal is to continue to learn about any potential risks and benefits of the drug now that it's being used by hundreds of thousands (or millions) of people.

The Vocabulary of Clinical Trials

Now that you know about the type of clinical trials, you need to understand the language of clinical trials, and what the various types mean for you.

> **Bet You Didn't Know**
>
> Even though a placebo is a "fake" treatment, it often has a powerful effect, called the *placebo effect*. Feeling better can occur after you receive the sham treatment, but is not related to any specific property of the sham treatment. It attests to the power of the mind over the body.

The gold standard clinical trial is a *double-blind, randomized, controlled trial*. What's that mean? *Double blind* means that neither the investigators (doctors or researchers) nor the patients know whether they are receiving the treatment under investigation, a placebo, or a different treatment.

Randomized just means that individuals signed up for the clinical trial are assigned to different *arms*, or treatment groups, within the trial, based on a completely random determination. This is usually decided via a computer program, although just flipping a nickel each time for each participant would work just as well. This is also called a *double-masked* study.

Controlled means that one group of participants receives the experimental drug, while another group (the control group) receives either the standard treatment for the disease or a placebo.

> **MedLingo**
>
> A **double-blind trial** means that neither the investigators (doctors or researchers) nor the patients know whether they are receiving the treatment under investigation, a placebo, or a different treatment. Usually, participants in these trials are **randomized**, or randomly assigned, to different **arms**, or treatment groups, within the trial. These trials are also usually **controlled**, meaning that one group is receiving the treatment under investigation and the other group is receiving a placebo or different treatment.

Getting into a Clinical Trial

Just because you've decided you're ready to join a clinical trial doesn't mean that it's ready to take you. You have to meet certain inclusion/exclusion requirements.

For instance, you might need to be a certain age, have certain blood sugar levels, *not* have certain complications, and not have other conditions—such as depression, arthritis, or cancer, which can interfere with study results.

Some studies want only men or only women; others are looking for a certain number of minorities, such as African Americans or Hispanics. Some might require that you not be on insulin, while others require that you be taking insulin. Every requirement is carefully planned to ensure that the investigators have designed the proper study to meet their requirements for information.

After you're accepted into a clinical trial, you'll primarily interact with a nurse, or clinical trial coordinator. This person will make sure that you turn up for regular appointments, track your information, see if you're okay with the proceedings, and generally keep you happy. Like a great aunt, he or she will also stay in touch even after the trial ends, to see if you have any other issues, complications, and so on.

You Are *Not* a Guinea Pig

Today's clinical trials are tightly controlled and regulated by both local and federal officials to protect you from harm and to make sure that you're aware of what you're getting yourself into.

The first step, even before you get involved, is for the doctor/group to receive approval from an *Investigational Review Board*, or *IRB*, which assesses the ethics and quality of the study to make sure that it is well designed. For instance, a clinical trial involving people who are seriously ill would not use a placebo; it would be unethical to deny patients medical care.

The study design is called the study *protocol*, a plan that describes who can participate in the trial; the schedule of tests, procedures, medications, and dosages; and how long the study lasts.

Then you have to provide *informed consent*. During this process, you learn the critical components of the clinical trial before deciding whether to participate. The medical staff involved in the trial should verbally explain what's involved, the possible side effects, and any potential dangers.

You should also have all this explained in a written document that is easy to read, written in your native language, and provides all key contacts.

This is not a contract; and even if you've signed an informed consent, you can decide to drop out of a clinical trial at any time. On the other hand, the investigator can force you to leave the study if you violate the protocol, for instance, by missing appointments.

MedLingo

An **institutional review board (IRB)** is a committee of physicians, statisticians, researchers, lay people living in the community, and others, who make sure a clinical trial is ethical and safe, and that the rights of study subjects are protected. An IRB must approve all clinical trials in the United States before they begin.

Informed consent refers to the process of learning the key facts about a clinical trial before deciding whether or not to participate.

The National Institutes of Health, which runs and funds hundreds of clinical trials every year, recommends that you ask the following questions before agreeing to participate in any trial:

- What is the purpose of the study?

- Who is going to be in the study?

- Why do researchers believe the experimental treatment being tested may be effective? Has it been tested before?

- What kinds of tests and experimental treatments are involved?

- How do the possible risks, side effects, and benefits in the study compare with my current treatment?

- How might this trial affect my daily life?

- How long will the trial last?

- Will hospitalization be required?

- Who will pay for the experimental treatment?

- Will I be reimbursed for other expenses?

- What type of long-term follow-up care is part of this study?

- How will I know that the experimental treatment is working?

- Will results of the trials be provided to me?

- Who will be in charge of my care?

Finding a Clinical Trial

It's pretty easy to find a clinical trial. Start with your doctors; they often know of trials in your area that recruit patients. Then go online. The NIH lists thousands of clinical trials, searchable by condition, at www.clinicaltrials.gov.

Other good sites include these:

- CenterWatch Clinical Trials at http://www.centerwatch.com/patient/studies/cat90.html. Type 2 diabetes in the search box. You'll see a listing of trials around the country and you can see if you qualify for any in your area.

◆ VeritasMedicine at www.veritasmedicine.com. VeritasMedicine.com is an online health resource focused on improving patient access to clinical trials and information about therapies in development for serious medical conditions. It contains a comprehensive clinical-trials database that matches patients to clinical trials based on information submitted confidentially.

The Least You Need to Know

◆ Clinical trials are an important process in the development of new treatments, methods of diagnosis, screening, and quality of life issues for diabetes and other medical conditions.

◆ There are several advantages and disadvantages of joining a clinical trial.

◆ All clinical trials must be approved by institutional review boards.

◆ There are several online sites to find information about diabetes-related clinical trials.

22

What Does the Future Hold?

In This Chapter

- New forms of insulin
- New medications beyond insulin
- Possible cures for diabetes
- First treatment for microvascular complications

If there's one advantage to the fact that type 2 diabetes has become epidemic in the Western world, it's that the sheer numbers of the scourge serve as an incentive to drug companies and medical device manufacturers to come up with new compounds and products to treat the disease.

And that's good news for you. It means a tremendous investment of time and money in diabetes by governments and private industry, new treatments coming onto the market, and the eventual possibility—perhaps even in your lifetime—of a cure.

Starting at the Top: New Insulins

We teased you a bit in Chapter 8 by telling you that researchers were working on new forms of insulin that didn't require shots. Well, the first ones should appear on the market within the next two years—maybe even sooner. These include the following:

◆ **Inhaled insulins.** Several are under development, but the one closest to reality is Exubera. Developed by Pfizer, Inc., Exubera is an inhaled insulin shown to work just as well as a short-acting injected insulin for both types of diabetes. Pfizer submitted its application for approval to the FDA in March 2005 and expected a decision later in 2005.

Even though this insulin is called "inhaled," it's actually delivered through your mouth, not your nose. You shoot a dry powder into your lungs using a device that looks like an asthma inhaler. The device "aerosolizes" the powder, that is, reduces it to very, very small particles that go deep into the lungs when you take a deep breath and hold it. From there, the insulin goes into the bloodstream and acts just like an injected short-acting insulin.

◆ **Oral insulin.** How about a form of insulin that you hold against your cheek until it's absorbed? It's not so far-fetched. Researchers are working on several forms of insulin that are absorbed by the mucous membrane in the mouth. One delivery mechanism under consideration comes from a form of seaweed!

Another form involves a liquid aerosol version of insulin that you spray into your mouth, where the mucous membranes in your cheeks, tongue, and throat absorb it.

◆ **Insulin in a pill.** Remember when we told you why there wasn't an insulin pill? Because both the acid in the stomach and the enzymes in the intestine would chew it up. Well, new formulations or coatings that protect the insulin molecule from stomach acid and intestinal enzymes are under investigation.

One form coats the insulin with a special gel enabling it to escape destruction in the stomach and intestines so that it can be absorbed into the bloodstream.

◆ **Insulin patch.** Patches are a well-known delivery system for hormones. Just think about the estrogen patch. Now researchers are working on a skin patch that would deliver a continuous low dose of insulin through the skin.

The patch actually requires a two-step process: In the first step, you apply an electronic adhesive patch powered by a tiny battery. It vaporizes cells on your skin, creating invisible openings (don't worry, it doesn't hurt). Then you stick on the patch.

Beyond Insulin: Hitting the Hormones

If insulin isn't an issue for you, don't despair. There's plenty coming down the pike for you, too. The following sections describe drugs under development that imitate the actions of certain hormones that play a role in insulin secretion and sensitivity.

Imitating Incretin

One approach focuses on *incretins*, hormones secreted by the intestine when you eat. Their major action is to increase insulin production by the pancreas, which prevents a spike in blood sugar after eating.

One incretin, called *glucagon-like peptide-1 (GLP-1)*, has two other actions. It prevents the pancreas from producing glucagon (recall that glucagon breaks down liver glycogen, the stored form of glucose), blunting any glucose rise after eating; and it slows the rate at which the stomach allows food to enter the intestine, further blunting any post-meal glucose rise.

A potential yet very important added bonus is that animal studies show that GLP-1 may help keep insulin-producing cells in the pancreas healthy. (Remember that one of the things that happens in type 2 diabetes is that these cells keep dying off, despite treatment to keep glucose levels near normal). Animal studies also show that GLP-1 may decrease appetite.

Finally, phase 3 studies (remember them from Chapter 21?) of a close cousin of GLP-1, called exenatide (see below) showed that patients who took this drug, actually lost weight. It's thought that GLP-1 and its cousin also work in the brain to decrease appetite. Researchers have known about GLP-1 for decades. The challenge of using it to treat type 2 diabetes is that after cells in the intestine release it, it stays around in the bloodstream for only a few minutes because an enzyme called *DPP-4* breaks it down very quickly.

MedLingo

Incretins are hormones secreted by the intestine when you eat. They prevent a spike in blood sugar after a meal by stimulating the pancreas to produce insulin. One, **GLP-1**, also prevents the alpha cells of the pancreas from producing glucagon (which releases glucose from the liver), and slows the rate of food exiting the stomach and entering the intestine, blunting the big surge of glucose into your bloodstream after eating. One problem is that GLP-1 only works for a couple of minutes before it is broken down by the enzyme **DPP-4**.

But thanks to the magic and genius of today's scientists, two approaches have been developed to get around this problem. One is to change the GLP-1 molecule so that DPP-4 can't break it down so quickly. One of these changed molecules (called exenatide) actually comes from the saliva of the beaded lizard, a close relative of the Gila monster.

Results from human studies lasting up to 82 weeks show good reductions in HbA1c levels using this approach. There is even some evidence that these drugs might suppress your appetite directly (at least, they did in animal studies), resulting in weight loss and thus improving insulin sensitivity. One potential drawback is nausea, but it eventually disappears. Another drawback is that the changed molecules of GLP-1 have to be injected. The good news is that the Federal Drug Administration approved exenatide (Byetta) in April 2005 for use in people with type 2 diabetes.

The second approach is to block the action of DPP-4. Early human studies with several DPP-4 inhibitors look promising. One advantage to this approach is that these new drugs can be taken orally; no needles!

All About Amylin Analogs

Amylin, a hormone secreted along with insulin from the beta cells also slows the digestion of food from the stomach and prevents the pancreas from secreting glucagon after eating. The FDA approved the first drug that mimics amylin, called pramlintide (Symlin), in March 2005 for use in type 1 and type 2 diabetic patients who also use insulin.

Two downsides are that it has to be injected and it can cause temporary nausea. But it seems to help manage blood sugar levels; a year-long study found that it reduced HbA1c levels and also led to weight loss.

Nonhormonal Medications on the Horizon

Numerous other medications are under development for people with type 2 diabetes who don't need insulin. These include the following:

- ◆ **PPARs** (peroxisome proliferator-activated receptors). There are at least two types of PPARs: gamma and alpha receptors. Existing TZDs (remember these?) affect the way your body metabolizes carbohydrates and fats, helping your muscles take in more glucose and thus decreasing insulin resistance and blood glucose levels, and they work on gamma receptors. But PPAR alpha receptors affect blood lipid levels, like cholesterol and triglycerides.

So researchers are developing medications that work on both receptors, a kind of cholesterol-and-glucose-lowering drug all in one. One drug in late-stage clinical trials, called muraglitazar, comes from Bristol-Myers Squibb and Merck.

It may also be the first drug to address the metabolic syndrome, a constellation of risk factors that leads to diabetes and heart disease.

Initial trials found that muraglitazar and a similar one under development by Astra Zeneca controlled blood sugar, cut triglycerides by over 30 percent, lowered LDL up to 20 percent, and increased HDL levels up to 15 percent.

◆ **K^+ (potassium) channel opener.** This compound, which relaxes blood vessels, doesn't even have a name yet. It's being developed as a treatment for both hypertension and diabetes. It affects production of insulin by beta cells, reducing their workload and, the theory goes, allowing them to rest more so they don't burn out. On the other hand, it also seems to improve glucose tolerance.

◆ **Orlistat.** This drug, already marketed under the trade name Xenical for the treatment of severe obesity, also appears to promote insulin sensitivity separate from weight loss. And that's just the indication (decreasing insulin resistance) for which its manufacturer, Roche Laboratories, Inc., asked the FDA. A decision was expected in mid- to late 2005.

Bet You Didn't Know

Someday, Botox (botulinum toxin) might be all you need to relieve the nausea, vomiting, and pain associated with diabetic gastroparesis. One small study of patients with type 1 diabetes found that a Botox injection (yes, the same stuff used to erase wrinkles) into the lining of the stomach through a tube inserted through the mouth significantly improved symptoms, including the time it took food to exit the stomach.

"P" is for Permanent: Implantable Insulin Pumps

Although we talked a lot about external insulin pumps in Chapter 9, we saved our discussion of internal insulin pumps for this chapter.

Currently, these pumps are approved only for use in the European Union and are used only for investigational use in the United States. Still, you might be able to gain use of one by signing up for a clinical trial, so here's what we do know about them.

Implantable pumps, about the size of the palm of your hand, require surgery, and they're considerably more expensive than external pumps (about $15,000 or more).

But they only require refilling every three months or so vs. the every three days or so required in external pumps, and the battery lasts about four years.

The insulin release is controlled via a hand-held, remote controlled device that can be set to release insulin continuously and provide boluses at mealtimes and bedtime. They're more commonly used in people with type 1 diabetes, and most of the studies on them have been conducted in this population.

But one study published in 1996 found that intensive insulin therapy with an implantable insulin pump had significant advantages over multiple insulin injections in reducing blood sugar ups and down, hypoglycemia, and weight gain, and, as might be expected from these changes, in improving aspects of quality of life.

The Possibility of a Cure

Part of the problem when it comes to finding a cure for diabetes is that researchers would like to find something that works for both those with type 1 and type 2—something that's very difficult to do. Nonetheless, work proceeds.

There are five main areas of focus when it comes to curing diabetes:

- ◆ Pancreatic transplantation
- ◆ Islet transplantation
- ◆ Engineered pancreatic beta cells
- ◆ The virtual pancreas
- ◆ Stem cells

Of Pancreases: Mine, Yours, Ours

Whole pancreas transplants are not some far-off-in-the-future dream; they're a reality today, primarily for people with type 1 diabetes. They are often performed along with a kidney transplant, and the results are pretty good, getting better every year.

But because the primary problem in type 2 diabetes is insulin resistance, not a total lack of insulin, the procedure is rarely performed in people with type 2 diabetes. According to the International Pancreas Transplant Registry, just 5 percent of pancreatic/kidney transplant recipients between 1997 and 2001 had type 2 diabetes. Reports of the eventual outcomes, however, suggest that after an initial spike in insulin resistance, the transplant resulted in a decrease in insulin resistance.

So given the emerging positive reports and the growing numbers of people with type 2, you can expect more doctors to try pancreatic transplants—if they can get the donors. While there were 2,022 pancreatic donors in 2004, there were 1,690 people on the waiting list for a pancreas only transplant, and 2,452 waiting for a pancreatic/ kidney transplant—about twice as many people needing the transplant as there were available donors.

Also, once the surgery is over, you have to take powerful drugs that suppress your immune system for the rest of your life, so your immune system doesn't reject, or attack, the donated organ(s).

Thus, whole pancreas transplants are currently reserved for patients who are either also receiving a kidney transplant or whose diabetes markedly affects their quality of life, for example, those with uncontrollable high blood sugars alternating with many episodes of hypoglycemia.

Islet Transplantation

Diabetes doctors and researchers are most excited about islet cell transplantation as a potential cure for diabetes. Currently, the way it works is that islet cells (in which insulin is produced) are isolated from whole pancreases in the lab, purified, and then injected into patients.

Although these transplants are still experimental, several studies are underway in people with type 1 diabetes to evaluate their success and identify any problems.

Again, powerful drugs to block the immune system are required after islet transplants. One advantage over whole-pancreas transplants, however, is that they don't require surgery. Instead, the purified islets are injected into the liver through a tube inserted through your bellybutton.

There are two problems with islet cell transplantation, however: it takes several donor pancreases to produce enough islet cells for transplantation and, as we mentioned earlier, sources of donor pancreases are limited. Also once injected, the islet cells seem to poop out over time.

One way around both of these problems is to take the islets from a donor pancreas and make them grow into more islets cells in the lab before transplantation. If that works, we'd need fewer donor pancreases and could inject more islet cells at one time. If the cells stop working, there would be an easy way to get more: Just grow them in the lab.

As you might imagine, researchers are working very hard on this approach.

Engineered Beta Cells

Along the same lines as islet cell transplantation, the idea behind engineered beta cells is to take other cells and change them into cells that can produce insulin in response to glucose. The newly created beta cells would then be implanted. This work is still very preliminary, occurring in the lab and in small animals.

Virtual Pancreas

No, this isn't some weird version of virtual reality. But a virtual pancreas, or actually, an artifical pancreas, is the goal of some very optimistic bioengineers. This approach differs from an implantable insulin pump because it would combine both the ability to deliver insulin with the ability to monitor glucose levels so that just the right amount of insulin is delivered.

These efforts are still in the early stages but a model implanted into the large veins of dogs has worked for a while.

Stem Cells

Stem cells are cells that have the potential to develop into almost any kind of more specialized cells, like brain cells, liver cells, red blood cells, white blood cells, intestinal cells, etc. They are present in early-stage embryos, and receive various signals to change into different cells and form organs.

However, some remain in the organs even after the organ is formed. One example is bone marrow (the middle part of certain bones), in which red and white blood cells continue to be produced from stem cells throughout a person's life.

Stem cells hold great promise in diabetes treatment and a possible cure, and researchers are investigating several possibilities for their use.

One approach, called *islet regeneration*, identifies the various biochemicals necessary to stimulate islet cell development from stem cells in a patient's own pancreas, and then gets those chemicals into the patient's pancreas. This approach, under investigation only in animals, could be used in people with both types of diabetes because, investigators say, both are related to a failure of pancreatic beta cells to respond to the needs of the body.

Another approach is to obtain stem cells from an external source, add these biochemicals to the stem cells in the lab so that they grow into new beta cells, and then transplant them into people with diabetes.

If successful, this technique could furnish an unlimited number of beta cells to cure an individual's diabetes. They might also be modified so that the patient doesn't need immune-suppressing drugs after transplant.

Treating Complications

In addition to finding ways to improve the way your body uses insulin and control glucose, researchers are also exploring ways to treat diabetes-related complications. Among the most promising are these:

◆ Drug manufacturer Eli Lilly is developing a drug called ruboxistaurin as the first treatment to address the various microvascular complications of diabetes to eyes, kidneys, and nerves. Currently in late-stage clinical trials, it appears to delay the development of vision loss in people with moderately severe to very severe nonproliferative diabetic retinopathy, and to provide some improvement in peripheral neuropathy and early kidney disease.

Ruboxistaurin works by blocking, or inhibiting, the action of the PKC b enzyme, which is thought to be at least partially responsible for the underlying process of microvascular damage that leads to microvascular complications. Stay tuned!

◆ As you learned in Chapter 17, macular edema is a major complication of diabetes. Although laser treatment stabilizes vision in most patients, some continue to get worse. Several small studies find that injecting steroids into the eyes of such patients can actually improves vision. Larger studies are underway.

◆ In Chapter 16, we mentioned that when glucose sticks to proteins in a process called glycosylation, the changed proteins cause some microvascular damage. So researchers are exploring compounds that slow the attachment of glucose to proteins. These compounds do a fabulous job of preventing the microvascular complications in animals, even when glucose levels in the blood remain high. One has been tested in humans but, unfortunately, the side effects were too dangerous for continued use. Still, the search continues for such a drug that doesn't have high levels of side effects.

The Least You Need to Know

- An inhaled form of insulin may be available as soon as 2006.

- Researchers are working on new drugs that can treat both hypertension and diabetes, or high blood lipids and diabetes, at the same time, as well as new drugs that attack type 2 diabetes in different ways.

- The quest for a cure for diabetes is alive and well, with artificial pancreases, stem-cell research, and pancreatic transplants leading the way.

- New approaches to treating the complications of diabetes are under investigation.

Glossary

acute-onset neuropathy (focal neuropathy)   A form of neuropathy usually involving just one nerve. Symptoms come on fast and it is usually quite painful.

adrenal glands   Glands that sit just above the kidneys and release adrenaline estrogen, progesterone, steroids, cortisol, and cortisone, and chemicals such as norepinephrine and dopamine.

adrenaline   A hormone secreted in times of stress that causes quickening of the heartbeat, strengthens the force of the heart's contraction, enables the lungs to take in more oxygen, and signals the liver to release extra blood sugar to help the body deal with great stresses.

albumin   A protein produced by the liver and found in plasma, the liquid part of the blood.

alpha and **beta blockers** (and **alpha/beta blockers**)   Drugs that partially block nerve signals to blood vessels and the heart in order to relax vessels and lower heartrate.

alpha cells   Cells in the pancreas that produce glucagon.

Alprostadil   A drug approved for the treatment of erectile dysfunction that is injected into the penis or inserted into the urethra in a suppository or capsule.

amino acids   The building blocks of proteins.

anatomy   The study of the parts and structure of the human body.

angina   The pain or squeezing sensation felt in the chest when the heart is not getting enough blood.

angiogram   A medical procedure in which contrast dye is injected into the blood stream enabling doctors (radiologists) to clearly see blood flow through many parts of your body.

angiotensin   A chemical that makes arteries contract.

angiotensin-converting enzyme (ACE) inhibitors   Medications used to treat high blood pressure by causing blood vessels to relax. They interfere with the production of angiotensin, a chemical that makes arteries contract.

angiotensin II receptor blockers (ARBs)   A high blood pressure drug that prevents angiotensin from stimulating cells to do their job.

arms   Different treatment groups within a clinical trial.

arteriovenous (AV) fistula   A form of venous access in which a surgeon connects an artery directly to a vein, usually in the forearm, to make the vein grow larger.

atherosclerosis   A condition that occurs when plaque, a substance composed of cholesterol, fibrous tissue, blood components, and calcium, builds up on the walls of arteries, stiffening and narrowing the arteries and interfering with blood flow.

atrial fibrillation   When the heart's electrical rhythm gets out of whack.

autoimmune disease   A disease that occurs when the immune system begins destroying normal, healthy cells. Autoimmune diseases include type 1 diabetes, lupus, multiple sclerosis, and rheumatoid arthritis.

autonomic nerves   Nerves, not under your conscious control, that receive signals from the central nervous system (CNS) and regulate certain functions that occur autonomically, such as breathing, digestion, heartbeat, and certain functions of smooth muscles in various organs controlling erections, urination, etc.

autonomic neuropathy   A form of neuropathy that affects the nerves in the autonomic nervous system.

AutonomicAV graft   A form of venous access in which the surgeon implants a synthetic tube under the skin in the arm to connect a vein and an artery.

beta cells   Specialized cells within the pancreas that make insulin.

bladder neuropathy   A form of autonomic neuropathy that occurs when the bladder nerves no longer respond normally to pressure.

body mass index (BMI)   A measurement used to classify people according to their weight (underweight, normal, overweight, obese) taking height into account.

calcium channel blockers   Hypertension drugs that help relax blood vessels.

capsaicin   A chemical that gives hot peppers their spiciness and is used in a topical cream to reduce pain.

cardiac stress test   A test that measures how well the heart works while the patient rides a stationary bicycle or walks on a treadmill.

cardiorespiratory fitness   A healthy state of heart and lungs resulting from regular aerobic workouts.

cardiovascular disease (CVD)   Diseases of the arteries.

cataracts   Cloudy lenses of the eye, generally age-related but more common in people with diabetes.

catheter   A thin plastic tube used in medical procedures and treatments.

central nervous system (CNS)   The part of the nervous system that consists of the brain and spinal cord.

Charcot joint (neuropathic arthropathy)   A form of neuropathy that occurs when the bones in the feet fracture because of repeated unnoticed trauma and the foot becomes misaligned.

clinical guidelines   Guidelines published by nonprofit organizations and government agencies that tell doctors the best way to prevent and treat certain conditions based on published research.

clinical proteinuria or macroalbuminuria   The loss of large amounts of protein into the urine, which is usually a sign of irreversible kidney damage.

clitoris   A female sexual organ, analogous to the penis.

co-insurance   The percentage of a medical fee a patient must pay; the insurance plan pays the rest.

compliant   Following suggestions by healthcare providers, e.g., taking your medications as directed.

congestive heart failure   The back-up of fluid in the lungs because the heart is too weak to pump blood normally.

continuous ambulatory peritoneal dialysis (CAPD)   The most common form of peritoneal dialysis, in which fluid is pumped into the abdomen and toxins the kidneys would normally remove but can't leach into the fluid. Then the fluid (and the toxins) are removed.

contraindicated   When a drug or treatment is not recommended because of some preexisting medical condition that might increase its negative side effects or cause other potential problems.

controlled clinical trial   A study in which one group of participants receive the treatment under investigation and the other group receives a placebo or different treatment.

coronary heart disease (or coronary artery disease)   A condition that occurs when the coronary arteries become narrowed or clogged by plaque consisting of cholesterol and other fat deposits, and can't supply enough blood to the heart.

corticosteroids   Anti-inflammatory drugs (normally secreted by the adrenal gland) injected into the back of the eye to treat macular edema.

cortisol   Hormone released under stress by the adrenal gland.

cranial neuropathy   A form of neuropathy that affects the nerves that move the eyeballs.

creatinine   A toxin that results from the breakdown of certain amino acids in the muscles. It is generally filtered out of the blood by the kidneys.

chronic disease   A disease that doesn't go away with treatment.

debride   To scrape away dead tissue.

deductible   The amount that must be paid by the insured toward health insurance costs before the health insurance company begins paying for services.

defibrillator   An electronic device that administers an electric shock to the heart through the chest wall in an attempt to restore the normal rhythm.

detached retina   A condition in which the retina pulls off from the back of the eye.

diabetic diarrhea   A form of autonomic neuropathy affecting the functioning of the small intestine.

diabetic neuropathy   The umbrella term for several conditions that affect the nervous system in people with diabetes.

diagnostic trials   Clinical trials designed to find new ways to diagnose diseases or conditions.

dialysis   A process by which a machine takes on the role of the kidneys, clearing the blood of toxins and other harmful substances.

dialysis solution   A solution used during peritoneal dialysis to pull wastes into the abdominal cavity, after which the fluid is drained out.

diaphragm   The muscular partition separating the abdominal cavity from the lung, or thoracic cavity.

diastolic pressure   Bottom marker of blood pressure reading that measures the pressure when the ventricle in the heart relaxes.

diuretics   Drugs that flush excess water and sodium from the body. Used to treat hypertension.

double-blind clinical trial   A trial in which neither the investigators (doctors or researchers) nor the patients know who is receiving the treatment under investigation.

DPP-4   An enzyme that breaks down the hormone GLP-1. DPP-4 is released from cells in the intestine and goes into the bloodstream.

dwell time   The amount of time the solution used in peritoneal dialysis typically remains in the abdominal cavity, typically four to six hours.

eclampsia   A toxic condition that occurs only during pregnancy and is characterized by protein in the urine, swelling, and hypertension that can lead to convulsions and possibly coma, if untreated.

electrocardiogram (EKG or ECG)   A test that measures and records the heart's electrical activity.

electrolytes   Dissolved salts in the bloodstream that are very important in maintaining homeostasis.

electromyographic examination   A test that measures the response of the muscles to an electrical shock. It is used to diagnose neuropathy.

endocrine system   The system of glands and hormones.

endocrinology A special field of medicine devoted to dealing with disorders of the endocrine system and hormonal disorders, including diabetes.

end-stage renal disease (ESRD) The point at which your kidneys can no longer clean out your blood, and you must go on dialysis three days a week to take over your kidney function.

epidemic A widespread outbreak of a disease affecting many people at one time.

epinephrine (adrenaline) Hormone released by the adrenal gland during stress.

erectile dysfunction Also called impotence, it refers to a man's inability to have and/or maintain an erection.

erythropoietin A hormone produced by the kidneys that increases the production of red blood cells.

exchange The process of filling the abdominal cavity with peritoneal dialysis solution and subsequently draining it during peritoneal dialysis.

exudates Deposits that result from leaking blood vessels in the eye.

fecal incontinence A condition in which stool leaks out; it occurs more commonly while sleeping.

fellowship Advanced training that doctors complete to specialize in a given field.

fetal hyperinsulinemia A condition in which the fetus gets too much glucose in his or her blood from the mother, increasing the fetus's insulin levels. This increases its fat cells, eventually resulting in a large baby and obesity and insulin resistance in childhood.

first-line treatments Drugs that are typically used first to treat a condition or disease because of their history of safety and effectiveness.

fluorescein angiography A procedure in which dye is injected in the arm and travels to the eye, enabling a doctor to better visualize any blood vessel problems and photograph them with a special camera.

focal laser A treatment for proliferative diabetic retinopathy in which a laser is used to seal leaking blood vessels and remove dead parts of the retina.

folic acid One of the B vitamins critical in the healthy development of a fetus.

foot drop A form of neuropathy that occurs when you can't pick up your foot because of a damaged nerve in the leg.

free radicals   By-products of normal chemical reactions.

fructosamine test   A test that measures how many blood glucose molecules are linked to albumin molecules in the blood, providing information on your average blood glucose level for the past three weeks.

funduscopy   An eye examination conducted using a special instrument called an ophthalmoscope to examine the retina.

gangrene   A condition that results when tissue doesn't get enough oxygenated blood and dies.

gastroparesis   A form of autonomic neuropathy affecting the stomach that prevents it from emptying normally.

generic drug   A drug that is the same as a branded drug, but is no longer protected by a patent. Thus, it may be produced by several drug companies, and is usually much less expensive than its branded cousin.

gestational diabetes   A condition called glucose intolerance that can develop during pregnancy when glucose levels are between normal and levels that would diagnose diabetes. The condition usually goes away once the baby is born.

gingivitis (periodontal disease)   A condition that results from infections caused by bacteria growing between your teeth and gums.

glands   Organs that release hormones.

glaucoma   A condition in which fluid doesn't drain normally from the eye. The build-up of fluid increases pressure in the eye, eventually destroying the optic nerve.

glomeruli   Clusters of tiny blood vessels in the kidneys that filter blood.

GLP-1   A hormone that increases insulin and decreases glucagon production by the pancreas, both of which prevent the liver from producing glucose. It also slows the rate of food exiting the stomach and entering the intestine.

glucagon   A hormone released from the pancreas when blood sugar levels drop.

glucose transporters   Proteins that ferry glucose molecules across the cell membrane.

glycated   The binding of glucose to protein products.

glycation   A process that occurs when glucose sticks to proteins and other cellular structures. The higher the glucose, the more glycation.

glycerol   One half of a glucose molecule produced when fat cells break down triglycerides.

glycogen   The storage form of glucose.

heart disease   Diseases of the heart, including heart attacks.

heart failure   When the heart muscle is too weak to pump blood throughout the body as well as it should.

hemodialyzer   An artificial kidney that filters the blood, returning clean blood to the body.

hemoglobin   The part of red blood cells that carry oxygen.

hemorrhages   Leaking blood vessels.

HgA1c   Also known as a glycated hemoglobin measurement, hemoglobin A1c, or simply as an A1C, it is a blood test that provides a picture of blood glucose levels for the past three or four months. High levels indicate problems controlling blood sugar for a long time before the test.

high-flux dialysis or **high efficiency dialysis**   A form of dialysis that removes larger molecules from the blood and takes about 25 percent less time than traditional hemodialysis.

high-risk individual   Someone who has a pre-existing medical condition, like hypertension, high cholesterol levels, diabetes, or heart disease, resulting in increased chances of becoming sick.

homeostasis   When the parts of the body and their functions are all in balance.

high-risk pregnancy   A pregnancy in which the mother and/or fetus have some underlying condition or problem that puts one or both of them at risk of complications.

hormones   Chemical messengers produced by glands in one part of the body that provide instructions to cells in another part of the body.

hyperglycemia   Higher-than-normal blood glucose levels.

hyperinsulinemia   Increased levels of insulin in blood because the pancreatic beta cells are producing too much insulin.

hypermagnesemia   Higher-than-normal magnesium levels in the blood.

hyperosmolar-nonketotic coma   Also called hyperglycemic nonketotic syndrome, it is a form of uncontrolled diabetes with extremely high blood glucose levels that occur without the presence of ketones in the urine.

hypertension   Blood pressure levels 140/90 or higher.

incretins   Hormones secreted by the intestine after eating, one of whose effects is increase insulin secretion.

indemnity plan   A plan in which medical services are paid for as they are used at the rate charged by the doctor or hospital.

induce   To artificially start labor.

informed consent   The process of learning the key facts about a clinical trial before deciding whether or not to participate.

institutional review board (IRB)   A committee of physicians, statisticians, and researchers, as well as lay people living in the community, and others, who make sure a clinical trial is ethical, safe, and that the rights of study subjects are protected.

insulin   A hormone secreted by the pancreas whose role is to maintain normal blood sugar levels, keep fat stored in fat cells, and make sure that protein is used to build muscles.

insulin analogs   Genetically engineered insulin products designed to change the way your body absorbs insulin.

insulin resistance   A condition that occurs when your body is unable to respond normally to insulin.

insulin sensitizer   A drug that improves how your body responds to insulin.

intermittent claudication   Muscle cramps in the legs that occur while walking and is the primary symptom of peripheral arterial disease (PAD), also called peripheral vascular disease (PVD).

intracavernosal injection test   A test for the cause of erectile dysfunction that involves injecting a medication into the penis to stimulate an erection.

intramuscular injection   An injection that goes into a muscle.

iris   The colored part of the eye.

islets of Langerhans   Structures in the pancreas containing alpha cells that produce glucagon and beta cells that produce insulin. They make up approximately 1 percent of the pancreas and are distributed throughout the organ.

islet regeneration   A process by which special chemicals are used to stimulate stem cells in the pancreas to grow into the alpha and beta cells that are normally contained in the islets of Langerhans.

isometric exercises   Exercises that involve the application of a force against an immoveable object, like sit-ups, push-ups, even pushing against a wall.

ketones   Chemicals that the body produces when it breaks down fat for energy.

lactic acid   A normal breakdown product of glucose metabolism. However, if there is not enough oxygen available in the body, dangerous levels of lactic acid can accumulate (*See* lactic acidosis).

lactic acidosis   A very serious condition that results when very high levels of lactic acid build up in the blood.

lancet   A small device used to prick the skin for blood tests.

libido   The desire to have sex.

lipids   Fats in the blood, primarily cholesterol and triglycerides.

macrovascular disease   Damage to the large arteries.

macula   A small spot in the retina where vision is sharpest.

macular edema   Fluid from leaking blood vessels that results in swelling of the macula.

Medigap insurance   An insurance policy that covers procedures, co-insurance, and other out-of-pocket costs that Medicare doesn't pay for.

membrane   The outer layer of a cell.

metabolic syndrome   A combination of conditions including obesity, high blood pressure, high glucose levels, high triglyceride levels, and low HDL cholesterol (the "good" cholesterol). Most people with the metabolic syndrome also have insulin resistance.

metabolize   The way in which the body breaks down a drug, usually in the liver, and clears the breakdown products of the drug from your body. The products are usually expelled through the kidneys by way of urine and sometimes through the intestines by way of stool.

microalbuminuria   When small amounts of albumin are excreted into the urine; a sign of early kidney disease.

microaneurysms   Sacs formed from bulging, weak blood vessels that occur during diabetic retinopathy.

microvascular complications or disease   Complications resulting from damage to the smallest blood vessels in the body, such as those found in the eyes, nerves, and kidneys.

monounsaturated fats   Vegetable oils and fatty acids whose molecular structure includes only one double carbon bond.

motor nerves   Nerves that carry signals from your brain and spinal cord to your muscles.

neonatologist   A doctor specially trained to take care of very sick newborns.

neovascular glaucoma   A condition that results from increased pressure in the eye, which could eventually lead to blindness.

neovasculization   The growth of new blood vessels on the surface of the retina or optic nerve.

nephrons   Small structures in the kidneys that contain the glomeruli.

nephropathy   A form of kidney disease occurring in people with diabetes.

nerve cells   A collection of fibers that transmit signals to and from the brain and spinal cord to other parts of the body.

nerve conduction tests   Tests that evaluate how well the nerves conduct sensation.

nervous system   The part of the body that provides sensory (what we feel), motor (moving muscles), and control mechanisms through a network of nerve cells.

nervous system inhibitors   Also called sympathetic nerve inhibitors, these drugs relax blood vessels by controlling nerve signals that cause blood vessels to constrict.

neuropathy   A disease of the autonomic and peripheral nerves. (*See* autonomic and peripheral neuropathies).

nitric oxide   A chemical that, among its many functions, relaxes blood vessels.

nocturnal penile tumescence test   Involves placing a band around the penis to test for involuntary erections during sleep.

nonproliferative diabetic retinopathy (NPDR)   Also called background retinopathy, this is a condition that occurs when blood vessels within the retina become weak and eventually begin leaking.

nonstress test   A test used during pregnancy, primarily in late pregnancy, to record the baby's heartbeat, providing a sense of the baby's health.

norepinephrine (noradrenaline)   Hormone released under stress by both the adrenal gland and certain nerve endings.

off-label use   When doctors prescribe an FDA-approved drug to treat a condition for which the drug has not been approved.

ophthalmologist   A medical doctor specially trained in diseases of the eye.

ophthalmoscope   A special instrument used to examine the retina.

optic nerve   The bundle of nerves that travels from the retina to the brain.

optometrist   An eye specialist who primarily performs routine eye exams and fittings for glasses and contact lenses.

orthotics   Devices used to support, align, prevent, or correct deformities or to improve the function of parts of the body, such as the foot.

osteoporosis   A condition in which the bones become weak and eventually break down, resulting in fractures.

oxidation   A process by which a form of oxygen becomes attached to a molecule, making it chemically unstable and resulting in cellular damage.

oxidative stress   The damage caused to molecules in your body from free radicals, byproducts of normal chemical reactions.

oxytocin   A natural hormone that causes the uterus to contract.

pancreas   An organ whose main function is to secrete enzymes into the small intestine to help digest food.

pancreatic islets   Small pieces of hormone-producing tissue within the pancreas.

peakless insulin   A form of insulin that has a steady effect on blood sugar, without any peak times of action. It usually causes less overnight hypoglycemia.

pedorthists, orthotists, or prosthetists   Individuals skilled in the manufacture of foot orthotics.

perinatologist   Specially trained physicians who treat women with high-risk pregnancies.

peripheral arterial disease (PAD)   Also called peripheral vascular disease (PVD). A condition in which the blood vessels in the legs narrow, causing pain while walking. If very severe, it may lead to amputation. It is associated with heart disease and stroke.

peripheral nervous system The part of the nervous system that consists of all nerves that branch out from the brain and spinal cord.

peripheral neuropathy A form of neuropathy that affects the nerves that go to the feet and, less often, to the hands, on both sides of your body. It first causes pain and then, as it progresses, numbness.

peripheral vascular disease (PVD) A catch-all term referring to problems caused by poor circulation due to clogged arteries in the legs.

peripheral vision The ability to see objects and movement outside of the direct line of vision.

physician network A group of physicians who agree to provide care for a certain payment.

physiology The study of how parts of the body function.

pilates A program of stretches and exercises designed to strengthen the core muscles of the back and abdomen.

pitocin A synthetic form of the natural hormone oxytocin, which causes the uterus to contract.

placebo A fake pill or treatment given to participants in clinical trials.

placenta A temporary organ connecting a mother with her growing fetus. It allows nutrients and other materials to pass from mother to baby.

plantar The ball of the foot, a common spot for diabetes-related foot ulcers.

plaque A substance composed of cholesterol, fibrous tissue, blood components, and calcium that builds up on the inside lining of artery walls.

podiatrist A specialist in the care of the feet.

polypharmacy Taking many medications at one time.

polyunsaturated fats Vegetable oils whose molecular structure has numerous double or triple bonds in a molecule.

postural hypotension A form of autonomic neuropathy that results in low blood pressure when standing up suddenly, leading to light-headedness and dizziness, and, if severe, fainting.

pre-eclampsia A problem that occurs during pregnancy, characterized by high blood pressure, fluid retention, and excess protein in the urine. It can lead to eclampsia.

pre-existing condition   A condition for which someone has received medical treatment in the past 12 months.

prehypertensive   A blood pressure reading of 120/80 to 139/89 mm Hg.

premiums   The amount of money paid for health insurance.

prescription compliance   Taking your medications as directed.

prevalence   Refers to how often a disease occurs within a given population.

priapism   An erection that lasts more than four hours and is usually painful.

proliferative diabetic retinopathy (PDR)   A condition that occurs when new blood vessels that are weaker than normal grow in the eye.

prophylactically   A medical treatment or procedure performed to prevent a disease.

quality-of-life trials   Clinical trials designed to find ways to improve the comfort and quality of life for people with chronic conditions.

quantitative sensory testing (QST)   A test that measures your sensitivity to temperature, touch, pressure, vibration, and pain.

randomize   To randomly assign participants in a clinical trial to different treatment groups.

reasonable accommodations   For people with diabetes, reasonable accommodations in the workplace are things such as breaks to eat or drink, take medication, or test your blood sugar levels and a private area in which to test blood sugar levels or take insulin.

receptors   Proteins within or on the outside of cells designed to bind to hormones and other chemicals produced within the body.

recombinant human insulin   A form of insulin that uses genetic engineering to turn bacteria into little insulin-producing factories.

rectum   The final part of the large intestine that controls bowel movements.

referral   Permission from the primary-care physician that is required before a patient can see a specialist.

residency   The years of training after medical school in a hospital setting spent by physicians before they can be licensed to practice medicine. Only one year is required for a license but almost all physicians take three or more years of training after medical school.

retina   The light-sensitive membrane covering the back wall of the eyeball that connects the images coming into the eye with the optic nerve.

reverse iontophoresis   A process in which a low electric current is used to move glucose through the skin for testing in a special meter.

rhabdomyolysis   A very rare condition that results in the breakdown of muscle tissue.

saturated fat   A kind of fat found in meat and other animal products. Solid at room temperature, it raises levels of blood cholesterol. Monounsaturated fats are generally the healthiest form of fats.

scatter laser treatment (panretinal photocoagulation)   A laser surgery used to destroy many different areas in the retina in order to prevent the signals that lead to new blood vessel growth.

screening trials   Clinical trials designed to find the best way to detect diseases or conditions.

self-monitoring of blood glucose (SMBG)   Home-testing of glucose levels using a glucose meter.

sensory nerves   Nerves that take messages from your body to your spinal cord and are then usually sent to the brain.

serotonin   A brain chemical that plays a role in depression and pain perception.

shoulder dystocia   When the shoulder of a large fetus gets wedged behind the mother's pubic bone, halting delivery.

sleep-disordered breathing (SDB)   Abnormal breathing patterns during sleep.

sleep apnea   When an individual stops breathing numerous times during the night for just a couple of seconds.

spina bifida   A birth defect in which the fetal spine fails to fuse early in development.

statins   A class of drugs used to treat high cholesterol levels.

starvation ketosis   A condition that occurs when the body begins breaking down fat for energy if there is not enough glucose to provide energy to muscle and other cells.

stem cells   Cells with the potential to develop into almost any kind of more specialized cells, like brain cells, liver cells, red blood cells, white blood cells, intestinal cells, etc.

stigma   A term used to describe the shame and social disgrace some people feel when they have a certain disease.

stress test   A test used during late pregnancy to record uterine contractions induced by medication.

stroke   Occurs when an artery in the brain becomes blocked, called an ischemic stroke, or bursts, called a hemorrhagic stroke.

subcutaneous injection   An injection into the layer of fat just beneath the skin.

sulfonylureas   A class of oral diabetes drugs that work by stimulating the pancreas to produce more insulin.

suppository   A capsule containing medication that is inserted into the urethra or rectum, where it releases the medicine.

sustained release   A medication in which the active ingredient is released very slowly.

systolic pressure   The top number of blood pressure, measuring the pressure when the left ventricle contracts.

testosterone   The major sex hormone in men.

transcutaneous electronic nerve stimulation (TENS)   A drug-free therapy that works by sending small electrical impulses from a small machine onto the skin that inhibits pain signals. This prevents the signals from reaching the spinal cord and, subsequently, the brain.

treatment trials   Clinical trials designed to test new drugs, devices, or other treatment methods, like radiation.

triglycerides   A form of fat carried in the blood stream and stored in fat tissue.

urethra   The tube through which urine passes out of the penis or vagina.

ultrasound   A test that uses sound waves to create an image of the inside of the body.

uterus   A hollow muscular organ in a woman's pelvic region that holds the developing fetus.

vascular access   A way to access the blood system.

vasodilators   Drugs that work as a kind of muscle relaxer for muscles in blood vessel walls, enabling the vessels to dilate or open wider.

venous catheter   A form of venous access in which a tube is permanently inserted into your neck, chest, or leg near the groin. It has two holes in its side so that blood can go out as well as in, and is used for hemodialysis when there is not enough time to prepare a vascular access.

ventricle   A heart chamber that pumps the blood out of the heart to the lungs (right ventricle) or to the rest of the body (left ventricle).

very low-density lipoprotein (VLDL)   Proteins that carry a lot of triglycerides on them.

visceral fat   Fat located around the organs inside the abdomen; it is deeper in the body than subcutaneous fat, which lies just under the skin. Visceral fat is associated more with insulin resistance than subcutaneous fat.

vitrectomy   Surgical procedure to remove bloodied vitreous gel through a small slit in the cornea and replace it with saline, or salt solution.

vitreous   The clear gel that fills the center of the eye.

Appendix B

Resources

There are many resources available if you'd like more information about type 2 diabetes and related topics. This section identifies books, websites, and organizations to help you broaden your knowledge.

Books

The American Diabetes Association. *American Diabetes Association Complete Guide to Diabetes: The Ultimate Home Reference from the Diabetes Experts.* New York: McGraw Hill Contemporary: 2002.

Beaser Richard S. *The Joslin Guide to Diabetes: A Program for Managing Your Treatment.* New York: Simon & Schuster, 1995.

Becker, Gretchen. *The First Year Type 2 Diabetes: An Essential Guide for the Newly Diagnosed.* New York: Marlowe & Co., 2001.

Bernstein, Richard K. *Dr. Bernstein's Diabetes Solution: The Complete Guide to Achieving Normal Blood Sugars Revised & Updated.* New York: Little, Brown, 2003.

Betty Crocker Editors. *Betty Crocker's Diabetes Cookbook: Everyday Meals, Easy as 1-2-3.* (Betty Crocker, 2003).

Brand-Miller, Jennie, et al. *The New Glucose Revolution Pocket Guide to Diabetes.* New York: Marlowe & Company, 2003.

Chase, H. Peter. *Understanding Diabetes.* Denver, CO: Children's Diabetes Foundation, 2002.

Drum, David and Terry Zierenberg. *The Type 2 Diabetes Sourcebook.* Los Angeles, CA: Lowell House, 2000.

Gruber, Carol. *Carol Guber's Type 2 Diabetes Life Plan: Take Charge, Take Care, and Feel Better Than Ever.* New York: Broadway, 2003.

Hiser, Elizabeth. *The Other Diabetes: Living and Eating Well with Type 2 Diabetes.* New York: Morrow Cookbooks, 2002.

Kaufman, Francine R. *Diabesity: The Obesity-Diabetes Epidemic That Threatens America—And What We Must Do to Stop It.* New York: Bantam, 2005.

McQuown, Judith H. *1,001 Tips for Living Well with Diabetes: Firsthand Advice that Really Works.* New York: Marlowe & Company, 2004.

Porter, Lance. *28 Days to Diabetes Control!: How to Lower Your Blood Sugar, Improve Your Health, and Reduce Your Risk of Diabetes Complications.* New York: M. Evans and Company, Inc., 2004.

Rosenthal, Sara M. *The Type 2 Diabetic Woman.* New York: McGraw-Hill, 1999.

Sauder, Christopher D., Richard R. Rubin, and Cynthia S. Shump. *The Johns Hopkins Guide to Diabetes for Today and Tomorrow.* Baltimore, MD: Johns Hopkins Press, 1997.

Valentine, Virginia. *Diabetes Type 2 & What to Do.* New York: McGraw-Hill, 1998.

Warshaw, Hope S. and Nancy S. Hughes. *The Diabetes Food and Nutrition Bible: A Complete Guide to Planning, Shopping, Cooking, and Eating.* Alexandria, VA: American Diabetes Association, 2001.

Whitaker, J. *Reversing Diabetes.* New York: Warner Books, 2001.

Websites

www.diabetesmonitor.com

Monitoring diabetes happenings everywhere in cyberspace, and providing information, education, and support for people with diabetes.

www.diabetesportal.org

A great starting point for all things diabetes, from information on insulin pumps to the latest news on diabetes. Also includes discussion groups and e-mailed newsletters.

www.helpingpatients.org

User-friendly information about pharmaceutical companies' patient assistance programs, for Medicare and other age groups.

www.ivanhoe.com/channels/p_channel.cfm?channelid=CHAN-100007

Diabetes-related articles and news, information on clinical trials and other diabetes tidbits on this easy-to-navigate and easy-to-understand site.

www.mendosa.com/diabetes.htm

Key diabetes-related Web resource for both types of diabetes run by freelance journalist David Mendosa, who has type 2 diabetes himself. Includes valuable information on diabetes-related equipment, medicine, lifestyle changes, and news.

www.nlm.nih.gov/medlineplus/diabetes.html

Government-sponsored and maintained portal that provides news as well as basic information about diabetes and diabetes-related complications.

www.togetherrx.com

The together Rx program that provides savings for income-eligible Medicare enrollees on more than 170 prescription medicines with one card.

Organizations

American Association of Diabetes Educators (AADE)
100 West Monroe, Suite 400
Chicago, IL 60603
Phone: 1-800-338-3633
Website: www.diabeteseducator.org

A multi-disciplinary organization of more than 10,000 health professionals dedicated to advocating quality diabetes education and care.

American Diabetes Association (ADA)
1701 North Beauregard Street
Alexandria, VA 22311
Phone: 1-800-342-2383
Website: www.diabetes.org

The leading educational, research, and advocacy diabetes organization.

American Dietetic Association (ADA)
120 South Riverside Plaza, Suite 2000
Chicago, IL 60606-6995
Phone: 312-899-0040
Website: www.eatright.org

Devoted to promoting optimal nutrition and well-being for all people.

Centers for Disease Control and Prevention (CDC) Division of Diabetes Translation
Mail Stop K-10
4770 Buford Highway, NE.
Atlanta, GA 30341-3717
Phone: 1-877-232-3422
Website: www.cdc.gov/diabetes

Provides information and materials on diabetes and works to reduce the burden of diabetes in the United States by planning, conducting, coordinating, and evaluating federal efforts to translate promising results of diabetes research into widespread clinical and public health practice.

Diabetes Action Research and Education Foundation
426 C Street, NE
Washington, DC 20002
Phone: 202-333-4520
Website: www.diabetesaction.org

Supports and promotes education and scientific research to enhance the quality of life for everyone affected by diabetes.

The National Institute of Diabetes and Digestive and Kidney Diseases (NIDDK)
1 Information Way
Bethesda, MD 20892-3560
Phone: 1-800-860-8747
Website: www.niddk.nih.gov

The government's lead agency for diabetes research, providing information clearing-houses and funding clinical research.

The Neuropathy Association
P.O. Box 26226
New York, NY 10117-3422
Phone: 212-692-0662
Website: www.neuropathy.org

Major Pump Manufacturers

Animas Corporation
590 Lancaster Avenue
Frazer, PA 19355
Phone: 610-644-8990
Website: www.animascorp.com

Dana Diabecare USA
541 Julia Street, Third Floor
New Orleans, LA 70130
Phone: 1-866-342-2322
Website: www.theinsulinpump.com

Deltec, Inc.
1265 Grey Fox Road
St. Paul, MN 55112
Phone: 1-800-426-2448
Website: www.delteccozmo.com

Medtronic MiniMed
18000 Devonshire Street
Northridge, CA 91325
Phone: 1-800-646-4633
Website: www.minimed.com

Nipro Diabetes Systems
10450 Doral Boulevard
Miami, FL 33178
Phone: 1-888-651-PUMP
Website: www.GlucoPro.com

Index

C

O

P

X–Y–Z